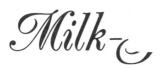 

MORE THAN 100 DAIRY-FREE RECIPES

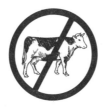

Ruby M. Brown

SALLY MILNER PUBLISHING

First published in 1991 by
Sally Milner Publishing Pty Ltd
17 Wharf Road
Birchgrove NSW 2041 Australia

© Ruby M Brown 1991

Production by Sylvana Scannapiego,
Island Graphics
Layout by Doric Order
Illustrations by Daphne Gooley
Photography by Andre Martin
Back cover photograph by Otto Knaus –
The Goulburn Studio
Typeset in Australia by Asset Typesetting Pty Ltd
Printed in Australia by The Book Printer

National Library of Australia
Cataloguing-in-Publication data:

Brown, Ruby M.

Milk-free cooking.

ISBN 1 86351 033 8.

1. Lactose intolerance – Diet therapy – Recipes.
2. Milk-free diet – Recipes. I. Title. (Series: Milner
healthy living cookbook).

641.563

Distributed in Australia by Transworld Publishers

Front cover:
Margaret Preston
Summer 1915
oil on canvas
51 x 51 cm
purchased 1920
Art Gallery of New South Wales

ABOUT THE AUTHOR

Ruby M. Brown is a qualified Home Economics teacher who has worked with students in all areas of this subject. She is a very skilled and dedicated teacher as well as a multi-talented culinary author.

This is her second book in the field of special diets. She has been able to help many people through her previous publication, *Wheat-Free Cooking*, which features more than 100 gluten-free recipes and an informative text on the subject. Ruby is the author of two very successful Country Kitchen books. *'Patonga' Country Kitchen* tells a story about her family and country property, nestled into the gentle slopes of the Southern Tablelands of New South Wales. In this book she compiled her family's traditional recipes created at her property which is now well known for its Country Kitchen Products. Her second book, *'The Explorer's' Country Kitchen* is a sequel, which draws together nutritious recipes representing many culinary styles.

She has written 12 text/workbooks for her students, who are inspired by her expertise in the culinary arts. She has written about aspects of Low-Cholesterol Diets, Healthy Eating, Meat Alternative Diets, and Special Diets. Ruby spends a great deal of her time writing about healthy eating for magazines and journals. She is well known as a guest speaker and for her work with people who have special dietary needs.

Ruby is a dedicated mother whose two teenage daughters share her culinary interests in this book.

She is a member of The Home Economics Association of Australia, The Home Economics Association of New South Wales, The Australian Capital Territory Home Economics Association, and The Australian Nutrition Foundation. She is a delegate to the triennial conferences of The Home Economics Association of Australia.

FOREWORD

It is a double pleasure and privilege to write this foreword for this latest 'special diet' work to come from Ruby Brown's talented culinary-art pen.

Firstly, I have witnessed first-hand the enthusiasm afforded her book *Wheat-Free Cooking* by sufferers of coeliac disease, who have attested to the variety and validity of her recipes.

This book, with its '100 dairy-free recipes', prepared using sound dietary and nutritional advice, will provide a similar and much needed resource for the many in the community unable to tolerate dairy products. Those who choose to restrict their dairy fat intake for other reasons will be delighted at the variety added to their daily fare by these recipes.

Secondly, I have also witnessed first-hand the author's dedication to integrity in the presentation of information and in the recipes she supplies — they are all 'tried and true'. Ruby has both a personal and professional interest and expertise in presenting the nutritional aspects of a special diet in a most tasty and appetising manner — so much for the myth that diet is 'die' with a 't'.

The recipes in all Ruby's books are easy to follow, nutritionally sound, tasty and guaranteed to work!

V. I. Feros,

Dr Viola I. Feros
(MB BS U of Q)

CONTENTS

ACKNOWLEDGEMENTS

I wish to express my most sincere thanks and appreciation to my family and others who have made many contributions to the publication of this book:

To my precious husband Kevin, for all the time, love and understanding you have expressed in our home while this book was being written. Without your untiring support for my work as an author, it would never have been possible.

To my two daughters, Maria and Angela-Mary, to whom I am devoted. Thank you for your contributions to this book. Your continued interest in the preparation of special diets in our home has been evidenced by the number of recipes you have helped me to compile.

To Mr Chris Black, Public Relations Manager of the Rice Growers' Co-operative Limited, Leeton, New South Wales my thanks for the information about Sunfarm Rice Bran.

To Alison and Michael Nicholls for your continued interest in critiquing my test-kitchen recipes. It is good to have friends who are so willing to sample my recipes and to know that the recipes fit into a low-cholesterol program for Michael's dietary needs.

To Doctor Viola Feros for her continued interest in my work as an author and for her words expressed in the Foreword to this book.

To Sally Milner and Marg Bowman, and the staff of Sally Milner Publishing for their continuing support for my work as one of their authors. It is a privilege to work with such a dynamic group of women.

This book is dedicated to my husband and two daughters. Without their continuing support for my work as an author, this book would not have been possible.

PREFACE

I do not in any way want to give the impression that dairy products are bad for all people and should not be consumed. There are, I know, nutritionalists who would support this theory. I would, however, like to address the fact that there are people in the community whose lives are improved if they delete milk and/or other dairy products from their diet. It is for these people that I recognised a need and have written this book. I trust some of the ailments brought on by their allergic reactions to dairy foods can be relieved by following the nutritious recipes in this book.

This book is also designed to help people who for their own reasons choose to follow a milk-free and/or dairy-free diet. There is now a fast-growing belief that the absence of dairy products from the diet greatly helps sufferers of asthma and rhinitis (nasal irritation). *Milk-Free Cooking* will interest any cooks who wish to add a repertoire of new recipes to their collection and want to widen their horizons and use products other than dairy foods, such as the readily available supply of soy products.

A special diet is a simple way to alleviate stress and trauma to the body caused by allergic and intolerant reactions to foods. People who were once willing to spend large amounts of money on drugs to heal their ailments are realising the value of diets which can control and alleviate their symptoms.

Dairy food intolerance is now widely recognised by the community and the medical profession. Some years ago, those who dared to mention a food intolerance or the need to follow a special diet were thought of as 'a little different'. Airline companies offer a variety of special diets for their passengers and large booksellers devote an entire section of their stores to books about special diets and food intolerances. The medical profession is showing increasing interest in the value of diets in the control of health problems. The continual stream of information that confronts us in the media must make people think deeply about food intolerance. One has to stop and think for only a short while to compile a long list of food allergies and intolerances. Reagents in foods can be in the form of chemicals, pesticides, artificial colourings, preservatives and naturally occurring proteins in legumes, milk, eggs and wheat.

Food allergies and intolerances are more common than most people realise. There are now reliable medical tests to determine whether a person's allergic reaction is to milk and/or other dairy products in the diet. If you fall into this group, or if for any other reason you want to remove these products from your diet, or choose to follow healthy eating practices, you will find many easy, interesting and varied recipes in this book.

I hope this book will prove it is possible to enjoy foods which exclude milk and/or dairy products from the diet and will encourage those who are facing a special dietary crisis in their lives.

Ruby M. Brown

INTRODUCTION

THE PRINCIPLES OF DIETARY HEALTH

A balanced diet should also be enjoyable. It should be made up of relaxed meals and snack times and should cater for personal tastes. It should also provide a balance of energy foods for body building and repair, and foods to regulate the body and keep it working smoothly.

Dairy products are an excellent source of protein, calcium, Vitamin A, and the Vitamin B group, for most people. If it is necessary or desired to follow a dairy-free diet, it is important to replace these foods with others that will provide the same nutrients. The removal of dairy products from the diet does not necessarily mean that you will not follow a nutritious diet.

Some people suffer an allergic reaction to cow's milk and its products. This can restrict these people to a small range of recipes and commercially prepared foods which contain no dairy products. Tofu and soy drink can be used in any recipe as substitutes for soft cheese and cow's milk. This book was written in the hope that it will provide people allergic to dairy products with a quick reference and a readily available supply of recipes to suit their dietary needs.

Many Australians eat unwisely. They eat too many foods which are not good for their body and too little nutritious foods. The majority of Australians eat far too much fat, sugar and salt, too little complex starch and fibre and drink too little water and too much alcohol.

Two very important health organisations — the National Heart Foundation and the Commonwealth Department of Health — fully recognise these problems and have developed guidelines to help to restore the balance to the Australian diet and lessen the possibility of our developing lifestyle diseases.

The National Heart Foundation's Dietary Goals

1. Decrease fat consumption to 30 per cent of total energy intake.
2. Substitute unsaturated fats for saturated fats where possible (so that saturated fats contribute no more than 10 per cent of total energy intake and polyunsaturated and monounsaturated fatty acids together contribute 20 per cent of total energy intake).
3. Achieve normal weight.
4. Decrease cholesterol intake to under 300 mg/day.
5. Limit alcohol intake (no more than 2 drinks/day).
6. Decrease salt intake.
7. Increase fibre intake.

In terms of food the National Heart Foundation advises people to:

1. Eat a wide variety of foods.
2. Keep to a healthy weight, if necessary by modifying energy intake and exercise patterns.
3. Eat fewer fatty foods.
4. Eat more bread, cereals, vegetables and fruit.
5. Eat fewer salty foods and less salt.
6. Drink less alcohol.

Australian Dietary Guidelines

The Eight Dietary Guidelines set out by the Commonwealth Department of Health are an important part of any dietary program.

Guideline 1 — Provide nutrition education and encourage all Australians to eat a nutritious diet.

Guideline 2 — Reduce the prevalence of obesity.

Guideline 3 — Decrease total fat consumption.

Guideline 4 — Decrease the consumption of refined sugars.

Guideline 5 — Increase the consumption of starch and dietary fibre, i.e., wholegrain cereals, vegetables and fruits.

Guideline 6 — Decrease the consumption of alcohol.

Guideline 7 — Decrease the consumption of salt.

Guideline 8 — Encourage breast feeding.

A wise guide to planning nutritious meals is the Australian Nutrition Foundation's "Healthy Diet Pyramid" which shows the proportions of each type of food that should be selected when planning nutritious meals.

The Healthy Diet Pyramid

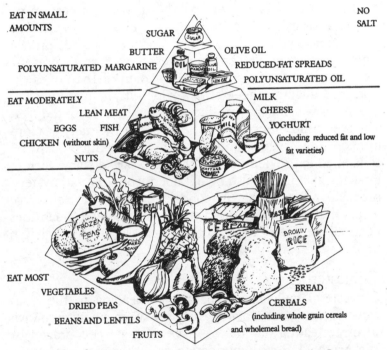

EAT IN SMALL AMOUNTS

NO SALT

SUGAR

BUTTER
POLYUNSATURATED MARGARINE

OLIVE OIL
REDUCED-FAT SPREADS
POLYUNSATURATED OIL

EAT MODERATELY
LEAN MEAT
EGGS   FISH
CHICKEN (without skin)
NUTS

MILK
CHEESE
YOGHURT
(including reduced fat and low fat varieties)

EAT MOST
VEGETABLES
DRIED PEAS
BEANS AND LENTILS
FRUITS

BREAD
CEREALS
(including whole grain cereals and wholemeal bread)

Reproduced with the permission of the Australian Nutrition Foundation Inc.

The recipes in this book are designed according to these guidelines. **They are low in fat, low in sugar, and contain no added salt or artificial preservatives or colours.**

Planning more enjoyable meals with these guidelines in mind will be possible by using the recipes in this book.

MILK-FREE/DAIRY-FREE DIETARY PRINCIPLES

Australian Food Standards Code

This code was written in 1987. It is published by the Commonwealth Government and is available from the Australian Government Publishing Service bookshops in each state. It will help you to understand more fully the labelling on food products.

Calcium Intake in the Diet

We have been made aware by the medical profession of the need for calcium in the diet, for the development and maintenance of healthy bones and teeth and proper functioning of nerves and muscles as well as to prevent the onset of osteoporosis (decalcification of the bones) in women. Calcium is generally provided in the diet by dairy products. When dairy products are removed from the diet, it is even more important to be aware of the daily calcium intake. Soy drinks and soya bean products can be consumed to provide some of the necessary dietary calcium intake. Calcium can also be obtained from salmon, oysters, broccoli and fresh fish. Almonds and cashews are also able to provide calcium in the diet but considerable quantities need to be eaten to reach the necessary daily calcium intake.

Cholesterol

Cholesterol build-up in the arteries leading to the heart can commence from a very early age when a person follows incorrect eating habits. We have all been encouraged by the National Heart Foundation to reduce our cholesterol level to a national average of below 5.5 mmol/L. The recipes in this book are designed with this in mind.

Complex Carbohydrates

Complex carbohydrates include all the polysaccharides present in food. They are composed of many monosaccharide units. These are the carbohydrates needed by the body for fibre. In Western countries complex carbohydrates tend to be forgotten and replaced by foods high in fat and sugar. It is best for the body's glucose to come from complex carbohydrates, rather than from straight sugar, as complex carbohydrate foods also supply other important nutrients. We should include more fruit, grains, breads, cereals and vegetables in our diet to obtain complex carbohydrates.

Daily Food Intake

The following is a suggested daily food intake. Remember to read labels carefully and select products with no dairy content.

BREAD AND CEREALS GROUP

Bread (preferably high fibre): 4 slices

Breakfast cereals (preferably high fibre, no added sugar): 1 serve

Other cereals (wheat, barley, rye, oats, rice, corn, millet, sorghum): 1 or more serves (depending on energy requirements)

FRUIT AND VEGETABLES GROUP

Vegetables (1 green vegetable, 1 white vegetable, 1 yellow vegetable): 3 serves

Fruit (fresh is best and eat at least 1 piece of citrus fruit each day for Vitamin C intake): 3 pieces

MEAT, FISH, POULTRY, LEGUMES GROUP

Lean meat, fish, lean poultry, legumes or eggs (2 to 7 eggs per week depending on cholesterol and fat levels): 2 serves

MILK AND DAIRY PRODUCTS GROUP

This has to be substituted with soy products.

Medical advice should always be obtained before undertaking a milk-free diet. This is especially important in young children and nursing mothers.

Daily soy drink requirements
Children: 600 ml
Older children and adolescents: 600-900 ml
Adults: 300-400 ml
Expectant and nursing mothers: 600-900 ml

Note: Soy products are available with both fat and sugar content reduced, it is preferable to use these. Some soy products are also available with added calcium. Take care to read the nutritional information on packages and select carefully to ensure the best nutritional requirements.

FATS AND OILS GROUP
No butter on a dairy-free diet.

Polyunsaturated margarine (milk-free varieties) (for low-cholesterol diets): 10 g

The amount indicated should be reduced if the fat intake is high in other areas as the total daily fat consumption should not exceed 30 per cent of the daily energy requirements. Note that Australian Dietary Guideline No 3 reminds us to reduce our fat consumption.

Dietary Fibre

Dietary fibre, originally described as roughage in the diet, is the term used to describe a group of substances which are mainly polysaccharides. Fibre is derived from plant cells (fruits, vegetables, cereals and nuts). The dietary fibre is the cell wall or structural framework of the plant cell, which holds the cell itself and the plant tissue together. It now includes pectins, lignins, gums and other non-digestible carbohydrates.

Dietary fibre cannot be digested or absorbed in the human gastro-intestinal tract but it stimulates the functioning of the colon. The fibre absorbs many times its weight in water and increases the volume of the stools passed, making for softer, easier elimination and the prevention of constipation. The inclusion of dietary fibre reduces the transit time of food through the gastro-intestinal tract and so aids the body in eliminating waste products. Dietary fibre is not a nutrient. It does not provide energy or build or repair tissues, nor regulate metabolic processes, but it plays a very important role in the way food affects body functions. It is credited with reducing the risk of some cancers, diverticulitis, haemorrhoids and varicose veins. The message to increase the intake of dietary fibre is one of the eight Australian Dietary Guidelines.

Fibre is very important when considering foods and planning healthy meals.

Fibre needed for healthy diets can be provided by wheat, barley, rye and oats. Polenta (also known as corn meal), maize meal, soya beans, and other beans such as kidney beans, cannellini beans, borlotti beans, garbanzo beans, mung beans, lentils, fresh fruits and vegetables, wholemeal flour and pasta, brown rice flour, rice, wheat, rice bran and oat bran, wheat germ, rolled rice flakes and ground rice all help to supply the much needed dietary fibre required by the body.

WAYS OF ADDING FIBRE TO YOUR DIET
1. Use soya bran, rice bran, oat bran, wheat bran or wheat germ. This can be added to cooking or sprinkled on breakfast cereals.
2. Use legumes in patties, soups, casseroles or stews.
3. Make your own muesli or have rolled oats for breakfast.
4. Use rolled oats in cooking.
5. Eat plenty of fresh vegetables and fruit. Remember — fresh is best.
6. Use cracked buckwheat kernels in cooking.
7. Use wholemeal rolled rice flakes.
8. Use wholemeal instead of white bread.

Dietitians
A major change of any kind in your diet should not be considered without a consultation with your doctor. Your

diet plan should be under the guidance of an experienced dietary consultant. Your local doctor or specialist can refer you to a dietitian. Dietitians can be contacted at major public hospitals, some community health centres or in private practice.

Dining Out

Remember, there is not the same social stigma attached to special diets in our society as there was some years ago. It is now socially acceptable, for the sake of your health, to be on a special diet. Don't be afraid to speak up. You will be the only person to suffer if you don't. Most chefs today have a good understanding of special diets and will be pleased to assist you with your needs. If it is at all possible, phone ahead and notify the chef of your special dietary requirements.

Labels

Always read the list of ingredients very carefully before purchasing. These points may help you when selecting products.

1. Read labels thoroughly and carefully.
2. Check the Manufactured Food Database, which is a list of ingredient information on manufactured foods, compiled by the Dietitians Association of Australia, PO Box 11, O'Connor, ACT 2601.
3. If you are in doubt, consult the manufacturer. They will welcome genuine enquiries for special diets.
4. Check with your doctor.
5. Check with your dietitian.

Manufactured Food Database

In 1989 the Dietitians Association of Australia (DAA) received a one year grant from the Department of Community Services and Health through its National Community Health Program to set up a databank of ingredient information on manufactured foods throughout Australia. The collated data will be printed in a standard format to be used by dietitians throughout Australia advising clients with special dietary requirements. In addition, specific lists of foods free of milk, egg, gluten and certain additives, etc., will be printed for members of the public requiring the information for medical reasons. These lists will be available from dietitians and doctors.

The Association hopes to continue the project with sponsorship from the food industry.

For further information on the databank, contact the Dietitians Association of Australia, PO Box 11, O'Connor, ACT 2601.

Meal Pattern
Sample daily meal pattern for a milk-free and/or dairy-free diet.

BREAKFAST
- Fruit or fruit juice (no added sugar).
- Wholegrain cereal with soy drink (lite).
- 2 slices high-fibre toast with a little polyunsaturated margarine (milk-free) with fruit spread (no added sugar), or other spreads (as desired).
- Tea and coffee substitutes are best, soy drink (lite), or water.

LUNCH (OR EVENING)
- Fish, lean meat, lean poultry, egg, tofu cheddar cheese alternative or peanut butter (no added salt).
- Salads and/or cooked vegetables (no oily dressings).
- 2 slices high-fibre bread with a little polyunsaturated margarine (milk-free).

- Fruit (fresh is best).
- Tea and coffee substitutes are best, soy drink (lite), or water.

MAIN MEAL
- Fish, lean meat, lean poultry and/or legumes.
- Potato, rice, corn and/or lentils (no fried foods).
- Vegetables (microwave or steam) and/or side salad (no added fat).
- Fruit (fresh is best). Forget the kilojoule-packed dessert!

MID-MORNING, MID-AFTERNOON AND SUPPER SNACKS
- Fresh fruit or vegetable sticks.
- Wholemeal crackers with tofu cheddar cheese alternative.
- Limit the amount of sweet biscuits and cakes.
- Healthy muffins are a wholesome snack.
- Soy drink (lite), fresh fruit juices (no added sugar), water, tea and coffee substitutes are best.

Travelling

When travelling, it is wise to carry a supply of your own food if space is available. Special dietary foods are not always available everywhere.

Most airlines offer a range of special diets. It is necessary to make a special diet request when you book your ticket. Food that leaves terminals other than those in Australia may not meet your dietary requirements. If you have a special dietary need, it is best to fly with the well-known carriers. It is a good idea to check the day before your flight, and when you check in, make sure your special diet has been ordered. Identify yourself to the flight attendant as you board the plane and indicate your special diet request. If you are travelling overseas you may be permitted to take some special dietary foods with you and bring some back into Australia. It is wise to carry an up-to-date letter from your doctor indicating your special diet as this can save time at customs, when travelling overseas.

Vegetarian Diets

People who follow a vegetarian diet do so for a range of reasons. There are varying degrees of vegetarianism and whatever form of vegetarian diet you choose, you should remember the need to provide your body with the eight essential amino acids. The eight essential amino acids are *isoleucine, leucine, lysine, methionine, phenylalanine, threonine, tryptophan* and *valine. Histidine* is also essential for children as their bodies are not able to make this amino acid fast enough for their growth rate. These building block proteins cannot be manufactured by the body and must be supplied in the daily diet. By eating a variety of vegetable foods such as grains, seeds, nuts, fruits and vegetables all the essential amino acids can easily be supplied. They are essential for growth and the maintenance of good health.

Vitamin B12 must also be included in the diet. It is found mainly in animal products. Vegans (those who consume no animal products whatsoever) have to rely on foods which have been fermented by micro-organisms to obtain Vitamin B12. Fermented soy sauce, miso (a fermented soya paste), tempeh (a fermented soya curd) and sauerkraut can provide some Vitamin B12. Mushrooms which have grown on a compost containing horse or chicken manure also contain Vitamin B12.

Lack of iron in the diet can also be a problem for the vegetarian. Meat and eggs are the main sources of iron in an omnivorous diet. When these foods are not consumed the iron intake must be found from dark green vegetables, beans, dried fruits, cocoa powder, molasses and/or fortified breakfast cereals. The absorption rate from these foods is not as high as that from animal products. The addition of folacin and Vitamin C in the diet helps the absorption of iron. See notes on Calcium Intake in the Diet on page 4.

GLOSSARY

HELPFUL INFORMATION FOR MILK-FREE DIETS

AGAR AGAR

Agar agar is a sea vegetable which is used as a gelatine substitute and can be used by those who wish to completely exclude animal products from their diet. It is used as a setting agent instead of gelatine for setting jellies and moulds, etc. It contains protein, iodine and iron and is available in the following forms:

Powdered — Agar agar is ground to a fine powder which resembles salt in colour and texture.

Flakes — This agar agar looks like small flakes of 'plastic'.

Strips — This agar agar is moulded into thin strips or long rectangular blocks. These forms of agar agar can be purchased at health food stores, and some supermarkets and chemist shops.

BEAN CURD

Bean curd is another name for tofu. Bean curd features on menus at Chinese and Japanese restaurants.

BISCUITS

Read labels carefully on commercial biscuits as they often contain dairy products.

BRAN

A nutritionally balanced, low-fat, high-fibre diet contributes to the prevention and control of diet-related diseases such as heart attack, diabetes and bowel disorders, including constipation and colon cancer. Wheat, soya, oat and rice bran are all excellent inclusions to add fibre intake to a diet. One relatively new bran on the market is Sunfarm Rice Bran. While oat bran has benefits related to cholesterol, and wheat bran has proven laxative benefits, the CSIRO's Division of Human Nutrition found that both benefits were available from Sunfarm Rice Bran. Rice bran also contains more soluble fibre than wheat bran and more insoluble fibre than oat bran. Marketed as 'the whole body bran' (because it is so broadly beneficial), Sunfarm Rice Bran is high in protein, mono and polyunsaturated fats, and dietary fibre. It contains the minerals calcium, magnesium, iron and zinc, and the vitamins thiamin, niacin, riboflavin and Vitamin E. It also contains the very smallest of the natural starches. The steaming process used to stabilise rice bran creates resistant starch which provides a slow and even conversion of carbohydrate to blood sugar. It is totally free of cholesterol and gluten, and is low in salt. It can absorb almost 5 times its bulk in liquid, making it an effective thickener for gravies, casseroles, sauces and soups. It lends rich, wholesome flavour and body to bread, biscuits, cakes, muffins and pies, and can also be sprinkled on breakfast cereal to add fibre.

BREAD
Wholemeal and high-fibre breads have the best nutritional value. Read labels carefully as a lot of commercial breads contain dairy products.

BUTTERMILK
This was traditionally obtained by draining the liquid from the churn as cream was churned into butter. It is not possible to purchase liquid buttermilk in this form, today. Cultured buttermilk is made by adding a safe bacterial culture to skim or part skim milk and is not a milk-free product.

CAROB
Carob is obtained from the pod of a Mediterranean tree. It is a nutritious chocolate-tasting food which contains calcium, phosphorus, iron, Vitamins A and B complex and its own natural sugar. Carob can be purchased in a powder form or as a chocolate confectionery alternative. In a chocolate confectionery form it has the advantage of not

containing caffeine or oxalic acid and is lower in fat content. Some carob confectioneries do not contain milk powder. It is important to read labels carefully before selecting.

CHEESE CAKES
A medium-firm tofu can be used instead of cream cheese in your favourite cheese cake recipe.

CHICKEN
When preparing chicken recipes, take care to trim all fat and skin from the flesh. This is particularly necessary when watching the fat intake in the diet.

COCONUT CREAM
Coconut cream is a product made from coconut flesh. It is a delicious mixture of fresh coconut and water which has been blended until very smooth. It is the consistency of thin custard and can be used as a substitute for cream in any recipe. It can also be blended with fruit juices, curries or desserts. It can be purchased in cans or heat treated packs from supermarkets or health food stores. It must be consumed with care when a low-cholesterol diet has to be followed as it contains saturated fatty acids.

COCONUT MILK
This is the liquid from the centre of the coconut. It has little nutritional value, being low in protein, vitamins and minerals. It is low in fat, having 220 kJ per 250 ml compared to coconut cream which has 795 kJ per 100 g. Coconut milk is also the term given to the liquid expressed after soaking desiccated coconut in boiling water. The fat and kilojoule content of this form of coconut milk will vary according to the pressure applied when extracting the liquid from the coconut.

COLD PRESSED OILS
Some people prefer to use cold pressed oils in their food preparation. These oils contain no artificial anti-oxidants. Some people wish to avoid the inclusion of anti-oxidants in their diet due to an intolerance to such additives. Some

cold pressed oils need to be kept in the refrigerator after opening. Olive oil has a high natural content of antioxidants which makes it quite safe at room temperature. All olive oil available in Australia is cold pressed. If you wish, you may substitute cold pressed oils for polyunsaturated vegetable oils when using the recipes in this book.

COOKING SPRAY
This is ideal for spraying cake tins and cooking dishes. Select a brand that is made from natural ingredients.

CREAM SUBSTITUTE
Tofu can be whipped in a blender with flavourings to make an excellent substitute for cream. See recipe for Tofu-Banana Cream on page 174.

CUSTARD
Substitute soy drink for cow's milk when making your favourite custard recipe.

DIP
A medium-soft or Japanese-style tofu can be substituted for cream cheese in any dip recipe. Dips are best made in an electric blender, food processor or electric mixer. Fresh tofu should be used. The flavour will develop if dips are made ahead of time and left in the refrigerator for several hours before serving.

EGG REPLACERS
Egg replacers can be purchased at health food stores. Some of these products are low in protein, fat, sodium, potassium and phenylalanine (an essential amino acid) and are high in calcium. Look for those products that are milk-free. They can be used to replace eggs in recipes. Follow the manufacturer's instructions for use. They have binding and raising properties which make them useful egg alternatives for special diets.

Egg replacers can be useful for:
1.   Those who have to reduce their cholesterol level.

2. Those who are allergic to eggs.
3. Those who do not wish to include animal products in their diet; and
4. Those on low-protein diets.

FRUIT SPREADS

Fruit spreads are so labelled when they contain no added sugar or artificial sweeteners. Read labels carefully and always buy reputable brands. Fruit spreads are classified apart from jams. To call a food a jam, it must contain either sugar or an artificial sweetening substance. Australian Dietary Guideline No 4 indicates a decrease in refined sugars is an important part of a dietary program, so if possible consume low-sugar jams or fruit spreads.

GREASING COOKING DISHES

Cooking spray and polyunsaturated oil can be used in place of butter or margarine for greasing cooking dishes, tins or trays. Check labels and use a brand made from natural ingredients.

ICE-CREAM

Soy drink can be substituted for milk when making ice-cream. Tofu can be blended with the soy drink to make a softer ice-cream. See recipe for Tofu Ice-cream on page 130.

LASAGNE

Slices of firm tofu can be added to a lasagne dish instead of a layer of cheese sauce. For added flavour, pour soy sauce over the tofu. Mashed tofu can be added to the meat sauce in your recipe. If you wish to make a cheese sauce, soy drink can be used instead of milk and tofu cheddar cheese alternative instead of cheese.

LEGUMES

Legume is the scientific name for pod-bearing plants. Legumes are the edible seeds and/or pods of the pulse family (peas, beans and lentils) and include black eye beans, borlotti beans, broad beans, cannellini beans, garbanzo beans, haricot beans, kidney beans, lima beans, mung beans, navy beans, soya beans, lentils, chick peas, snow peas and peanuts. Legumes add fibre to the diet. We are reminded in Australian Dietary Guideline No 5 to increase the consumption of starch and dietary fibre in our diet.

LENTILS
Lentils are a variety of legume. They are the dried seeds of many varieties of Lens esculenta plants. They are suitable for inclusion in a healthy diet.

MAIZE MEAL
Maize kernels are ground coarsely to produce this meal. It is coarser than polenta (corn meal).

MALTODEXTRINS
Maltodextrins are used in commercial products for sweetening and stabilising. They are prepared by drying a mixture of dextrins and oligosaccharides and reducing sugars obtained from the partial hydrolysis of starch. The starch used could be wheaten starch or potato starch.

MAYONNAISE
Soft tofu or soft Japanese-style tofu is best to use when making mayonnaise. You will get a very smooth result if you use an electric blender, food processor or mixer. It is important to use very fresh tofu to make mayonnaise. If you wish to reduce the fat content, you can leave the oil out of a mayonnaise recipe when using tofu and still get a smooth, creamy result. Read labels carefully on commercial products to see whether dairy products are included. Homemade low-fat recipes are always best. See recipe for Tofu Mayonnaise on page 175.

MEAT
The recipes in this book use lean, good quality cuts of meat with all visible fat removed, in keeping with National Heart Foundation guidelines for healthy eating.

MICROWAVE-SAFE BOWLS
Microwave-safe bowls should be used when cooking food in the microwave oven. Some plastics, polished wood,

some metal containers and dishes with metal trims are not suitable. Consult your microwave instruction book if you are in doubt.

MILK SHAKES

Cold soy drink can be used instead of cow's milk to make milk shakes. For extra body and flavour, soy drink powder can be added. Use two teaspoons of soy drink powder to each one cup of soy drink.

MISO

Miso is a paste prepared from fermented soybeans. Other grains, such as wheat, buckwheat, barley or rice are added to the soybeans, causing variations in flavour and colour. The longer the fermentation, the darker the colour and the richer the flavour. Miso is available in several colours ranging from brownish black ('Mugi Miso' or 'Kome Miso') to a light golden colour ('White Miso'). 'White Miso' is very popular as the flavour is light savoury and not too over-powering. Sea-salt is sometimes added. Miso contains the concentrated nutrients of soybeans with the addition of Vitamin B12, due to the fermentation process. Miso is useful for those with poor digestive systems as it is easily digested. It can be used to flavour soups, added to drinks and sauces, to casseroles and stews, and meat and vegetable dishes. It can be added to boiling water to make instant stock. It can be purchased from some supermarkets, health food stores and oriental grocery stores.

MONOSODIUM GLUTAMATE

Monosodium Glutamate (MSG) or Additive 621, is used to enhance the flavour of protein food. It stimulates the taste buds and has the effect of increasing the appetite for more of the foods flavoured with MSG. For most people it is an extra source of sodium. It has been blamed for some unpleasant side effects such as palpitations and dizziness experienced by some people. It must be remembered that MSG occurs quite naturally in some foods. Mushrooms, tomatoes, tomato juice, tomato paste, tomato purée, strong cheeses, yeast, vegetable or meat extracts and some wines are high in MSG. When a packaged food contains MSG it must be so marked.

NIGARI
Nigari is the solid residue left after the salt extraction process from sea water. It is a commonly-used 'setting-agent'. When it is added to hot soy drink, curds and whey form, thus forming the initial process of making tofu. Nigari can be purchased from health food stores and oriental grocery stores. It is best stored in a dry, airtight container.

OKARA
Soybeans which have been soaked and cooked for the production of soy drink and tofu are puréed to make okara. It is a nutritious food with great versatility in cookery. It can be used when making cakes and loaves, biscuits, desserts and puddings, and pâtés. When it is to be used in cooking, it is best roasted to impart a sweet, nutty flavour. Roasting it in a hot oven also dries it out and allows it to keep longer. It can be kept in an airtight container in the refrigerator or frozen for several weeks. It will add fibre and protein to the diet.

PASTAS
Buy wholemeal pastas whenever possible. These help to add fibre to the diet. Read labels carefully to ensure the purchase of milk-free pastas.

POLENTA
Polenta is the Italian name for corn meal. This is ground from the maize kernel. It is suitable for coarse breads. Polenta is excellent for adding fibre to the diet, as well as some protein, vitamins and iron.

QUICHES
Tofu can be used in place of milk in a quiche. This adds flavour and will thicken the quiche as it cooks. Soy drink can also be used instead of milk.

SALT SKIP
'Salt Skip' is a low-salt raising agent. It may be used in place of baking powder. It can be purchased at health food stores.

SAUCES
Read labels carefully for inclusion of dairy products before buying sauces of any kind.

SAUSAGES
Some sausages contain dairy products in powdered form. Always check for inclusion of dairy products before purchasing. Remember that most sausages are high in fat and should be used sparingly in any diet. Some butchers, if requested, will prepare sausages from lean meats, with no added salt or seasonings.

SEMOLINA
This is the granular starchy product obtained from the endosperm of hard wheat. Semolina flour is the fine floury part of the endosperm. Semolina will add fibre to the diet as well as providing some vitamins and minerals.

SHORTENING FOR COOKING
Recipes in this book are made with polyunsaturated vegetable oil, peanut oil, olive oil, or milk-free polyunsaturated margarine. You can choose your own shortening to suit your individual needs. Keep the quantity down to a minimum, wherever possible, as we are reminded in Australian Dietary Guideline No 3.

SHOYU SAUCE
This sauce is made from a mixture of fermented soybeans and wheat. It has a slightly milder flavour than tamari. Shoyu sauce is available in a reduced salt form. It can be purchased from health food stores and oriental grocery stores.

SOYA BEANS
Soya beans are available in forms such as miso, soybean oil, okara, soy crunch, soyeroni (soy pasta), soy flour, soy

grits, soy drink, soy sauce, tempeh, tofu and textured vegetable protein (TVP) as well as in the whole-bean form. Soya beans provide versatility and economy when planning meals. They are an excellent source of low cost protein. Vegetarians have been enjoying the benefits of soya beans for many years. They are a plant food which contains all the essential amino acids found in meat. They also contain fibre, Vitamin A, B group vitamins, iron, zinc, potassium, phosphorus and calcium. Vitamin C is available from sprouted soya beans. They are now being recognised in wider dietary circles for their nutritional value, economy, versatility and their use as a substitute for dairy products for allergy sufferers.

In Australia, the most popular dried soya beans are about half a centimetre long and are a creamy colour. They are extremely tough and require special treatment to make them edible and digestible. For this to take place, they must be soaked for several hours before cooking. The liquid in which the beans have been soaked will be bitter and is thrown away. The cooking process softens the soya beans thus allowing them to be digested and the nutrients to be more readily absorbed by the body.

Dried and canned forms are very popular due to their long shelf life. Canned soya beans are already soaked and cooked and can be used immediately they are opened. Soya bean can be purchased fresh, dried or canned from supermarkets, delicatessens and health food stores.

SOYA-COTTAGE CHEESE
This product resembles the cow's milk version of cottage cheese. It is made from a firm tofu and has a crumbly appearance. It has a stronger flavour than the mild cow's milk form. It is useful in making desserts and dips. It can be purchased from health food stores. If you find it difficult to purchase 'soya-cottage cheese', you can use sieved soft tofu as a substitute in recipes.

SOY CRUNCH
This product has the texture of coarse flour, being made from a mixture of soy chips, wheat germ, millet, polenta

and linseed. It may also be used as a thickening agent in soups and casseroles. It can be used instead of breadcrumbs to coat food for shallow frying. Remember Australian Dietary Guideline No 3 to decrease fat consumption in the diet, so avoid fried foods where possible.

SOY DRINK
Soy drink can be used in place of milk in recipes when a milk-free diet is chosen. It is sometimes referred to as soy 'milk', because it is used instead of dairy milk. It is necessary to read labels carefully when planning a milk-free diet as there are some soy drinks on the market that are combined with dairy drinks.

Soy drink is made from soya beans. Soya beans are soaked in water for several hours. The soaking liquid is drained and discarded and the beans are ground. The beans are cooked for approximately two hours and the liquid extracted from the beans is strained. Unflavoured, it has a sweet, nutty taste.

The nutritional value of soy drink is similar to dairy milk. It has approximately the same amount of protein and B vitamins and more iron than cow's milk. The calcium content is about one-fifth that of cow's milk. Some commercial products are fortified with extra calcium to bring them to the same level as cow's milk. Soy drink has an added bonus of containing no cholesterol and less fat than cow's milk. It can now be purchased in a 'lite' form which has a fat content of less than one per cent.

Soy drink is of great benefit to those who have allergic reactions to cow's milk. Some infants cannot tolerate cow's milk, but have been known to flourish on soy formulae. These can be obtained from chemist shops.

Heat treated packs of soy milk from a wide variety of brands and flavours can now be purchased from health food stores and supermarkets. The chemical compositions do vary, so choose the brand which best suits your needs.

Soy drink is also available in a dried powder form. Careful reading of labels is necessary as some brands contain lactose which would be a problem to an allergic lactose sufferer.

Soy drink can be substituted for cow's milk in all recipes. It has a slight disadvantage of being more expensive than cow's milk. To compensate for this, some of the soy drink can be replaced with water in cooking.

SOYERONI
This is a pasta made from soy flour and semolina. It can be substituted for other pastas such as macaroni. It can be purchased from health food stores, delicatessens and supermarkets. Check labels for dairy products.

SOY FLOUR
Soy flour is made by grinding soya beans. It has a fine texture and a very strong and bitter taste when raw. This bitter flavour will be reduced with cooking. Soy flour contains no gluten and is therefore best used in combination with other flours, to help bind the product. It will add protein, calcium, phosphorus and potassium to the diet. Soy flour can be used to thicken soups and casseroles. It can be purchased from supermarkets and health food stores.

SOY GRITS
Roasted soybeans are ground to a coarse meal to make soy grits, which are like cracked wheat in texture. They can be added to casseroles, soups, cakes and rissoles, as well as other recipes. They can be purchased from supermarkets and health food stores.

SOYBEAN OIL
This oil has a mild flavour and odour and is popular for all forms of cooking, as well as salad dressings and salads. It can be purchased from supermarkets and health food stores.

SOY SAUCE
This sauce is made from fermented soya beans. It has slight nutritional value with small amounts of proteins, vitamins and minerals being present. It is necessary to

check labels carefully to ensure a pure, naturally brewed product. A salt-reduced variety is now available.

SOY YOGHURT
This yoghurt, made from soy drink, has a light curdy texture and a 'bean' flavour. If you have not tasted it before, be prepared for a flavour unlike that of yoghurt made from cow's or goat's milk. It can be purchased from health food stores.

TAHINI
This creamy paste is made by grinding sesame seeds and adding sesame or peanut oil to make a product similar to peanut butter. It is a nutritious addition to dips and spreads, sauces and dressings. It is important to restrict the use of oily foods on a low-fat diet.

TAMARI
This is pure soy sauce. It is a natural food with rich flavour, and does not contain wheat. It can be used in any way that soy sauce would be used. A low-salt variety is now available and can be purchased from health food stores.

TAPIOCA
This is the starch prepared from the root of the cassava plant. The starch paste is heated to burst the granules. It is then dried in globules resembling sago. It adds fibre when included in the diet.

TEMPEH
A mould culture holds together a firm cake of partially cooked soybeans to make a product known as tempeh. It has a chewy texture and can be easily sliced or chopped because of its fibre content, and can be used in many recipes such as soups, casseroles, rissoles and salads. With its slightly more distinctive flavour than tofu, it is best used in savoury recipes. It is nutritionally important for its Vitamin B12 and protein content, iron and some calcium. This is of great importance to vegetarians as Vitamin B12 is usually found in animal foods. The fermentation process used to make tempeh brings about

the production of Vitamin B12. Tempeh is an easily digested food, like tofu, with the beans having been precooked and further tenderised by the fermentation process. Fresh tempeh can be stored in the refrigerator for one week or it can be frozen. It can be eaten when fresh, in its 'raw' state, however the best flavour will be developed during cooking. Tempeh can be purchased from supermarkets and health food stores.

TEXTURED VEGETABLE PROTEIN (TVP)
TVP is a product for the meat alternative diet which adds nourishment and texture to many recipes. It is made by removing the oil from soya beans, then taking out the carbohydrate. The remaining protein slurry is then forced through a spinning device with small holes. The protein comes out of the holes in fibres which are washed, flavoured, coloured and spun into different textures. TVP can also be made from oil seeds, including peanut, cottonseed, sunflower and safflower. It is high in protein and low in fat. It unfortunately can have a high salt content and contain artificial flavours and colours. It is available from supermarkets and health food stores and can be purchased in a wide variety of brands and flavours. Some may contain dairy products, so read labels carefully.

TOFU
This is commonly known as 'bean-curd'. It is made by curdling the mild white 'milk' of the soya bean. It is one of the world's most versatile protein foods. It is extensively used in Chinese and Japanese cooking. It is also known as 'soybean cheese', because it is made from soy 'milk'. It has been a protein staple in parts of Asia for over two thousand years. Tofu is enjoying a rise in popularity in Australia as it is a highly nutritious food that is easily digested, low in fat and free of cholesterol and is economical and versatile. It is rich in protein, vitamins, especially B vitamins, and minerals, especially calcium and iron. As it is low in kilojoules it makes a good substitute for meat, eggs and/or cheese in recipes. Its bland flavour

allows it to be used in cakes and desserts and even ice-cream. Silken tofu is available in heat-treated packs and is best suited to making desserts. Chinese and Japanese tofu varies according to the curdy texture and setting agents used. Dried tofu is also available and can be reconstituted by soaking in water. Fresh tofu is packed in water to retain its freshness. It should be pale greyish white in colour with a sweet 'bean' smell. It will keep, while sealed, in the refrigerator for 2 weeks, or it can be frozen. Tofu can be purchased from supermarkets and health food stores.

TOFU CHEDDAR CHEESE ALTERNATIVE
This product closely resembles the cow's milk version of cheddar cheese. It is made from organic tofu, canola oil, calcium caseinate (protein), sea salt, citric acid, natural cheddar cheese flavour, soy lecithin, guar gum with added annatto food colour. It is also available in a low sodium variety for those who wish to restrict sodium intake. It is free of cholesterol, free of lactose and low in saturated fat due to the use of canola oil. It can be purchased from some supermarkets and health food stores.

WATER
Water is an essential substance to life, second only to air in its importance. All drinks contain some water. The best way to supply the body with its need for water is to drink at least eight glasses (2 litres) of fresh, clean water every day.

WHERE TO BUY MILK-FREE AND DAIRY-FREE PRODUCTS
Leading retailers are now including a wider range of dairy-free products on their shelves. Most health food stores also carry a wide range of products. If your local supermarket does not carry the lines you require, ask. Most large retailers are happy to be educated about special dietary products. Remember your supermarket owner is not an expert in special dietary needs.

WHITE SAUCE
Follow the basic recipe and use soy drink instead of milk. Sieved, soft tofu can be added to help thicken a sauce. Substitute Tofu Cheddar Cheese Alternative in place of cheese.

WHOLEMEAL FLOUR
The recipes in this book use wholemeal flour. Wholemeal flour adds fibre and nutrients to the diet. You may use white flour instead of wholemeal flour if you wish.

MEASUREMENTS AND CONVERSION TABLES

All measurements in this book are made using Australian Standard metric cup and spoon measures.

1. Standard fractional measuring cups are used for measuring dry ingredients. They come in four sizes: 1 cup, ½ cup, ⅓ cup and ¼ cup. All measurements are level cupfuls.

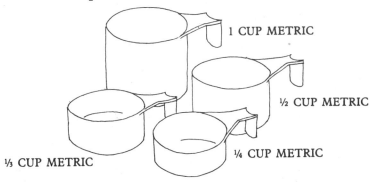

1 CUP METRIC

½ CUP METRIC

⅓ CUP METRIC

¼ CUP METRIC

2. A metric cup measure is used for measuring liquid ingredients. Equivalences are:

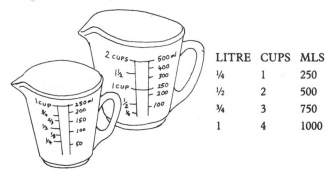

LITRE	CUPS	MLS
¼	1	250
½	2	500
¾	3	750
1	4	1000

All metric cup measurements are read at eye level with the cup on a level surface.

3. Metric spoons are used for measuring dry or liquid ingredients. They generally come in a set of four: ¼ teaspoon (1.25 ml), ½ teaspoon (2.5 ml), 1 teaspoon (5 ml) and 1 tablespoon (20 ml). All spoon measurements are level spoonfuls, unless otherwise stated.

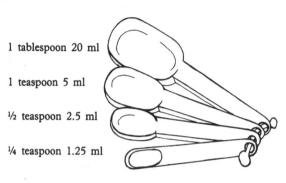

1 tablespoon 20 ml

1 teaspoon 5 ml

½ teaspoon 2.5 ml

¼ teaspoon 1.25 ml

Commonly Accepted Metric Conversions Used in Cookery
DRY WEIGHT

METRIC		AVOIRDUPOIS
15 grams		½ ounce
30 grams		1 ounce
60 grams		2 ounces
90 grams		3 ounces
125 grams		4 ounces (¼ pound)
155 grams		5 ounces
185 grams		6 ounces
220 grams		7 ounces
250 grams		8 ounces (½ pound)
280 grams		9 ounces
315 grams		10 ounces
345 grams		11 ounces
375 grams		12 ounces (¾ pound)
410 grams		13 ounces
440 grams		14 ounces
470 grams		15 ounces
500 grams	(0.5 kilogram)	16 ounces (1 pound)
750 grams		24 ounces (1½ pounds)
1000 grams	(1 kilogram)	32 ounces (2 pounds)
1500 grams	(1.5 kilograms)	3 pounds
2000 grams	(2 kilograms)	4 pounds

LIQUID

METRIC	IMPERIAL
30 millilitres	1 ounce
100 millilitres	3 ounces
150 millilitres	5 ounces
250 millilitres	8 ounces
300 millilitres	10 ounces (½ pint)
500 millilitres	16 ounces
600 millilitres	20 ounces (1 pint)

Oven Temperatures

It is very difficult to advise on exact oven temperatures. Different makes of stoves give different results at the same temperature setting. You are the best judge of the heat settings of your own stove for the particular product you are cooking. The cooking time for a product will also vary greatly between different kinds of stoves. Fan forced ovens in the newer stoves have reduced cooking times considerably. Also, many of the foods in this book can be successfully prepared in a microwave oven. In this case cooking times will be greatly reduced, and further variations in cooking time are possible depending on the heat setting chosen. The following chart should help.

	ELECTRICITY		GAS	
	Celsius	Fahrenheit	Celsius	Fahrenheit
Very Slow	120	250	120	250
Slow	150	300	140-150	275-300
Moderately slow	160-180	325-350	160	325
Moderate	190-200	375-400	180	350
Moderately hot	220-230	425-450	190	375
Hot	250-260	475-500	200-230	400-450
Very hot	270-290	525-550	250-260	475-500

Microwave Oven Cooking Times

A 600 watt microwave oven has been used when making recipes in this book. Microwave cooking times will vary with different wattage ovens, type of container, temperature and volume of ingredients, etc. There is no exact way to predict cooking times. A good rule to remember is always to undercook rather than overcook.

31

RECIPES

Title pages to sections indicate which recipes are milk-free, wheat-free, egg-free, low-fat and low-sugar.

Title pages also indicate the suitability for cooking in a convection and/or microwave oven. Suitability for freezing is also indicated.

MILK-FREE PRODUCTS

At the time of printing, all manufacturers' prepared products used in these recipes were milk-free. As manufacturers change the composition of their products from time to time, it is always necessary to check ingredients on prepared products carefully before purchasing.

Abbreviations used in this book:

C — Celsius
F — Fahrenheit
g — grams
oz(s) — ounce(s)
kg — kilogram
lb(s) — pound(s)
cm — centimetre
" — inch

* Registered Trade Marks
  Kellogg's (Aust) Pty Ltd
  Authorised user

† Trade Mark

SOUPS AND STARTERS

	MILK-FREE	WHEAT-FREE	EGG-FREE	LOW-FAT	LOW-SUGAR	CONVECTION	MICROWAVE	FREEZER
STARTERS								
Cucumber Rings	•	•	•	•	•			
Hommus	•	•	•	•	•			
Pineapple Mushrooms	•	•	•	•	•			
Smoked Salmon Dip	•	•	•	•	•			
Spinach Pâté	•	•	•	•	•	•	•	
Soya-Cottage Pâté	•	•	•		•			
SOUPS								
Cauliflower Soup	•	•	•	•	•	•		•
Pumpkin Vichyssoise	•	•	•	•	•	•		•
Tomato Soup	•	•	•	•	•	•	•	•
Tuna Soup	•	•	•	•	•	•		•
Zucchini Gazpacho	•	•	•	•	•	•	•	•

CUCUMBER RINGS

These Cucumber Rings can be served as an hors d'oeuvre, entrée or as an accompaniment to a salad.

INGREDIENTS

1 long green cucumber
200 g (7 ozs) soft tofu, mashed
½ banana, peeled and cut into small cubes
1 tablespoon lemon juice
2 tablespoons finely chopped walnuts
½ cup well drained, finely chopped pineapple
(in natural juice)
2 shallots, finely chopped
1 tablespoon finely chopped fresh mint
2 tablespoons finely chopped fresh chives
(to sprinkle on top)
nutmeg (to sprinkle on top)

METHOD

1. Wash cucumber. Score skin and cut cucumber into rings approx. 3 mm (¼″) thick. Cut at least 12 rings.
2. Place remaining ingredients except chives and nutmeg into a medium sized mixing bowl and mix well.
3. Place approx. 1 tablespoon of mixture onto each cucumber ring.
4. Sprinkle with finely chopped chives and nutmeg.
5. Arrange on a large flat serving dish.

HOMMUS

Hommus is made and eaten as a pâté or a dip. This recipe is an easy version as it uses fresh, cooked beans instead of the traditional garbanzo beans, which require several hours of cooking. A 245 g can of beans (no added salt) can be used instead of fresh beans. Hommus can be made the day before it is required and the topping added just before serving. It can be served with dry crackers or toast, as desired.

INGREDIENTS
1½ cups cooked beans
½ cup tahini
juice of 1 lemon
2 cloves garlic, peeled and crushed
1 small onion, peeled and cut into small dice
1 stick celery, finely chopped
1 tablespoon olive oil (for topping)
1 tablespoon lemon juice (for topping)
1 tablespoon finely chopped fresh mint (for topping)

METHOD
1. Blend beans, tahini, lemon juice, garlic and onion in the bowl of an electric food processor or blender.
2. Stir celery into Hommus.
3. Place into a serving bowl.
4. Just prior to serving, mix together olive oil, lemon juice and mint. Pour over Hommus.

Serves 12 as a pâté or dip.

PINEAPPLE MUSHROOMS

Mushrooms are an excellent source of nutrition. They are low in fat and high in fibre. This recipe can be used as an entrée or as a vegetable accompaniment to a main course.

INGREDIENTS
12 medium sized mushrooms
1 x 200 g carton tofu cottage cheese
½ cup well drained, finely chopped pineapple pieces
    (in natural juice)
2 shallots, finely chopped
1 tablespoon finely chopped fresh mint
freshly ground black pepper (as desired)
2 tablespoons finely chopped chives
    (to sprinkle on top)
paprika (to sprinkle on top)

METHOD
1. Wash mushrooms and carefully remove stalks. Set mushrooms aside.
2. Finely chop stalks and place into a small mixing bowl.
3. Add remaining ingredients except chives and paprika to bowl and mix well.
4. Place approx. 1 tablespoon of mixture into the cavity of each mushroom.
5. Sprinkle each mushroom with chives and paprika.

Serve 3 mushrooms as an entrée or 2 mushrooms as a vegetable accompaniment.

SMOKED SALMON DIP

Smoked salmon makes a lovely dip. The dip can be served with wholemeal crackers or wholemeal toast (milk-free).

INGREDIENTS
100 g (3½ ozs) cooked smoked salmon, flaked
1 x 100 g can smoked salmon spread
¼ cup finely chopped fresh parsley
1 tablespoon Sunfarm rice bran
2 teaspoons lemon juice
½ teaspoon dried basil leaves
¼ teaspoon dried sage leaves
½ teaspoon dried mixed herbs
1 clove garlic, peeled and crushed

METHOD
1. Blend all the ingredients in the bowl of an electric food processor or blender (or mix together by hand).
2. Store in a covered container in the refrigerator until required.

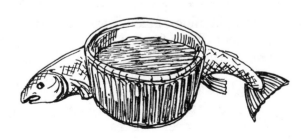

SPINACH PATE

This recipe combines vegetables and meat to make a very tasty pâté.

INGREDIENTS
1 bunch fresh young spinach
250 g (8 ozs) bacon, finely chopped
  (all skin and fat removed)
750 g (1½ lb) lean minced steak
2 onions, peeled and finely chopped
2 cloves garlic, peeled and crushed
1 teaspoon powdered rosemary
½ teaspoon dried thyme
¼ teaspoon cayenne pepper
2 tablespoons gelatine
3 tablespoons water
1 cup soy drink

METHOD
1. Prepare a 2 litre (3 pt) fluted mould by lightly oiling.
2. Wash spinach. Remove white stalks. These can be reserved and used as a vegetable if desired.
3. Chop leaves. Place into a steamer and steam until tender.
4. *Convection Cookery.* Place bacon into a large flat pan. Cook for approx. 5 minutes over a moderate heat. Add mince, onion, garlic, herbs and pepper and cook for a further 10 minutes approx. or until meat is tender.
   or
   Microwave Cookery. Place bacon onto absorbent paper on a flat microwave-safe plate. Cover with absorbent paper. Microwave on high for 1 minute. Stir bacon and microwave on high for

a further 1 minute. Transfer cooked bacon to a large microwave-safe bowl. Add mince, onion, garlic, herbs and pepper and cook for a further 5 minutes approx. or until meat is tender.

5. Blend spinach and cooked ingredients in an electric food processor or blender or rub through a sieve or Mouli. It will be necessary to blend the ingredients in portions. Pour into a large bowl and stir well.
6. Place gelatine into a small bowl. Stir in water. Allow to stand for 3 minutes.
7. *Convection Cookery.* Place soaked gelatine into a small saucepan. Stir over a gentle heat until liquid boils.

or

Microwave Cookery. Place soaked gelatine into a small microwave-safe bowl. Microwave on high for 30 seconds and stir. Microwave on high for a further 20 seconds or until liquid boils.
8. Pour liquid into bowl with blended ingredients. Add soy drink and stir well. Pour into prepared mould.
9. Refrigerate until firm.
10. Turn out onto a flat plate to serve.

Serves 6-8.

SOYA-COTTAGE PATE

This pâté is made from crisp fresh vegetables.

INGREDIENTS
1 tomato
2 tablespoons gelatine
1/3 cup cold water
500 g (1 lb) soya cottage cheese
1 carrot, peeled and finely grated
1 small zucchini, finely grated
1 small head broccoli, finely chopped
1/2 teaspoon dried mixed herbs
1/4 teaspoon dried coriander
1/4 teaspoon paprika
1 clove garlic, peeled and crushed
freshly ground black pepper (as desired)
1 teaspoon concentrated vegetable stock
1 tablespoon finely chopped fresh mint
lettuce (for serving)

METHOD
1. Lightly oil a medium sized mould or basin.
2. Place tomato into boiling water for 1 minute. Remove skin and finely chop.
3. Place gelatine into a small saucepan. Stir in water. Allow to stand for 5 minutes. Stir over a gentle heat until mixture boils.
4. Blend all the ingredients except lettuce in the bowl of an electric food processor or blender (or mix together by hand).
5. Pour into prepared mould.
6. Cover and refrigerate overnight.
7. When ready to serve, turn out of mould onto a bed of lettuce.

Serves 6.

CAULIFLOWER SOUP

This soup is a combination of wholesome vegetables. It has no added fat or salt.

INGREDIENTS

1 small cauliflower, chopped
1 large potato, peeled and chopped
1 medium sized onion, peeled and chopped
1 clove garlic, peeled and crushed
4 cups vegetable stock
1 teaspoon concentrated vegetable stock
½ teaspoon dried dill tips
½ teaspoon dried sage leaves
1 teaspoon dried mixed herbs (Italian variety)
½ cup soy drink powder

METHOD

1. Place vegetables, stocks and herbs into a large saucepan.
2. Cook with the lid on until vegetables are soft.
3. Blend portions of vegetables and liquid in the bowl of an electric food processor or blender or rub through a sieve or Mouli.
4. Stir in soy drink powder.
5. Reheat and serve as desired.

Serves 6.

PUMPKIN VICHYSSOISE

This is a delicious pumpkin soup made from a selection of wholesome fresh vegetables.

INGREDIENTS
1 kg (2 lb) pumpkin, peeled and chopped
2 large onions, peeled and chopped
4 medium potatoes, peeled and chopped
1 clove garlic, peeled and crushed
4 cups vegetable stock
1 teaspoon dried mixed herbs (Italian variety)
1 teaspoon dried dill tips
¼ teaspoon dried coriander
¼ teaspoon nutmeg
1 cup soy drink powder

METHOD
1. Place vegetables, stock, herbs and spices into a large saucepan.
2. Cook over a gentle heat with lid on until vegetables are soft.
3. Blend cooked vegetables, stock, herbs, spices and soy drink powder in the bowl of an electric food processor or blender. It will be necessary to blend the vegetables in portions.
4. Return to saucepan and reheat before serving.

Serves 6.

TOMATO SOUP

INGREDIENTS

1 x 850 g can peeled tomatoes (no added salt)
1 small onion, peeled and cut into small cubes
1 carrot, peeled and cut into small cubes
1 potato, peeled and cut into small cubes
1 cup vegetable stock
2 tablespoons tomato paste (no added salt)
1 teaspoon dried dill tips
¼ teaspoon dried cumin
¼ teaspoon dried sage
¼ teaspoon dried cardamom
¼ teaspoon dried marjoram
1 tablespoon finely chopped fresh parsley
½ cup soy drink powder
¼ cup warm water

METHOD

1. *Convection Cookery.* Place vegetables, stock and tomato paste into a medium sized saucepan. Cook with the lid on until vegetables are soft.

   or

   Microwave Cookery. Place vegetables, stock and tomato paste into a medium sized microwave-safe bowl. Cover with vented plastic wrap. Microwave on high for approx. 6 minutes or until vegetables are soft.

2. Blend vegetables and liquid in the bowl of an electric food processor or blender or rub through a sieve or Mouli.

3. Stir in herbs.

4. Reheat to just below boiling point.

5. Blend soy drink powder with warm water. Stir into soup. Do not boil or soup will curdle.

Serves 4.

TUNA SOUP

This is a thick nutritious soup that can be served before a main meal or used as a mini meal.

INGREDIENTS
1 fillet fish (approx. 500 g [1 lb])
2 cups water
1 x 425 g can tuna (no added salt or oil)
1 x 425 g can peeled tomatoes (no added salt)
1 onion, peeled and chopped
1 medium sized carrot, peeled and chopped
½ cup white wine
½ cup soy drink powder
2 teaspoons curry powder (as desired)
1 teaspoon mustard
1 stalk celery, finely diced
juice of ½ lemon

METHOD
1. Place fish fillet into a large saucepan. Add water and cook over a gentle heat until fish flakes easily.
2. Remove bones and skin from fish. Blend fish and liquid in the bowl of an electric food processor or blender. Return to saucepan.
3. Remove and discard any bones present in tuna and flake with a fork. Add tuna and juice to saucepan.
4. Blend tomatoes, onion, carrot, wine, soy drink powder, curry powder and mustard in the bowl of an electric food processor or blender. Pour into saucepan with fish stock. Add celery.
5. Stir over a gentle heat until heated through.
6. Just before serving, stir in lemon juice. Do not boil or soup may curdle.

Serves 6.

ZUCCHINI GAZPACHO

Gazpacho can be served hot or cold as desired at the beginning of a meal in place of a thick soup.

INGREDIENTS
3 large tomatoes
1 teaspoon olive oil
1 large onion, peeled and finely chopped
½ red capsicum, seeded and finely chopped
1 stick celery, finely chopped
2 cups finely grated zucchini
½ teaspoon dried sweet basil
¼ teaspoon dried coriander
½ teaspoon dried mixed herbs
freshly ground black pepper (as desired)
1 clove garlic, peeled and crushed
1 cup water
1 teaspoon concentrated vegetable stock
2 tablespoons finely chopped fresh parsley

METHOD
1. Place tomatoes into boiling water for 1 minute. Remove skins and finely chop.
2. Place oil into a large saucepan. Add onion and cook until soft.
3. Add tomato and remaining ingredients.
4. *Convection Cookery.* Cook over a gentle heat with lid on for approx. 5 minutes or until vegetables are tender.
or
   Microwave Cookery. Place into a large microwave-safe bowl and microwave on high for approx. 5 minutes or until vegetables are tender, stirring occasionally.

Serves 6.

MAIN COURSES

	MILK-FREE	WHEAT-FREE	EGG-FREE	LOW-FAT	LOW-SUGAR	CONVECTION	MICROWAVE	FREEZER
CHICKEN								
Apricot Chicken Breasts	•			•	•	•		•
Chicken with Broccoli	•	•	•	•	•	•	•	
Chicken Curry	•	•	•		•	•	•	•
Chicken with Plum Sauce	•	•	•	•	•	•		•
Chicken Satay	•	•	•	•		•	•	
Crispy Chicken Pieces	•	•		•	•	•	•	•
Chinese Chicken	•	•	•	•	•	•	•	•
FISH								
Fish Kebabs	•	•	•	•	•	•	•	
Fish Cakes	•			•	•	•	•	•
Fish Lasagne	•		•		•	•	•	
Fish and Spinach Rice	•		•	•	•	•	•	
Trout with Almonds	•		•	•	•	•	•	
Tuna Loaf	•	•		•	•	•	•	
Tasty Salmon Mould	•	•	•		•	•	•	

MEAT

	MILK-FREE	WHEAT-FREE	EGG-FREE	LOW-FAT	LOW-SUGAR	CONVECTION	MICROWAVE	FREEZER
Beef Meatballs	•	•	•	•	•	•		•
Spaghetti Bolognese	•		•	•	•	•	•	•
Ham Potato and Ham Croquettes	•			•	•	•	•	
Lamb Lamb Pies	•		•	•	•	•		•
Lamb and Vegetable Pies	•		•	•	•	•		•
Pork and Lamb Surprise	•	•	•	•	•	•	•	•
Veal Osso Bucco	•	•	•	•	•	•	•	•
Veal in Red Wine	•	•	•	•	•	•		•
Veal and Vegetable Loaf	•	•		•	•	•		•

MEAT ALTERNATIVE

	MILK-FREE	WHEAT-FREE	EGG-FREE	LOW-FAT	LOW-SUGAR	CONVECTION	MICROWAVE	FREEZER
Beans Borlotti	•	•	•	•	•	•	•	•
Bean Casserole	•	•	•	•	•	•	•	
Butternut Rice	•	•	•	•	•	•	•	
Carrot Quiche	•				•	•		
Nut Loaf	•	•			•	•	•	•
Pita Pizzas	•		•	•	•	•	•	•
Potato and Celery Pie	•				•	•	•	
Soya Bean Pizza	•		•		•	•		•
Soya Patties	•	•		•	•	•		•
Vegetable-Mango Patties	•			•	•	•	•	•
Wholemeal Patties	•			•	•	•		•

APRICOT CHICKEN BREASTS

This delicious recipe uses chicken breasts, stuffed with apricot filling. It is an excellent way to use chicken in a low-fat diet. Apricot Chicken Breasts can be served with vegetables, rice and/or salad as desired.

INGREDIENTS

APRICOT FILLING
¼ cup finely chopped dried apricots
¼ cup boiling water
2 tablespoons tempeh
¼ cup crushed Kellogg's* All-Bran†
2 tablespoons finely chopped celery
1 tablespoon finely chopped fresh parsley
freshly ground black pepper (as desired)

CHICKEN
4 boned chicken breasts (all skin and fat removed)
½ cup crushed Kellogg's* All-Bran†
1 tablespoon finely chopped fresh parsley
freshly ground black pepper (as desired)
1 egg white, lightly beaten
olive oil (for cooking)

METHOD

APRICOT FILLING
1. Mix ingredients together and refrigerate for half an hour.

CHICKEN
1. Pound chicken breasts gently, taking care not to break the flesh.
2. Spread each chicken breast with Apricot Filling.
3. Roll up and secure with a poultry skewer or toothpicks.
4. Mix together All-Bran, parsley and black pepper.

5. Brush each chicken roll with lightly beaten egg white.
6. Toss chicken rolls in crumb mixture.
7. Heat a little oil in a non-stick frying pan. Cook chicken until golden brown, turning frequently. It is important to cook until chicken is cooked right through. This will be approx. 20 minutes.

Serves 4.

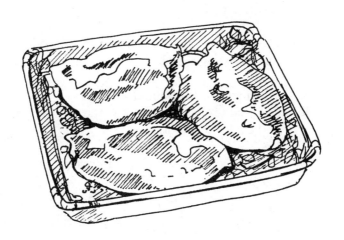

CHICKEN WITH BROCCOLI

Meals that are quick and easy to prepare and are at the same time nutritious are always favourites in my kitchen. This recipe can be served on a bed of cooked brown rice or wholemeal pasta.

INGREDIENTS
500 g (1 lb) small new potatoes
500 g (1 lb) chicken fillets (all skin and fat
removed), cut into small cubes
500 g (1 lb) broccoli flowerettes
¼ cup soy sauce (low-salt, wheat-free)
2 tablespoons dry sherry
¼ teaspoon dried marjoram
½ teaspoon dried basil
freshly ground black pepper (as desired)
6 whole cloves
2 bay leaves
1 cup mung bean sprouts

METHOD
1. Preheat oven to 200°C (400°F) for convection cookery.
2. Prepare a 2 litre flat convection or microwave-safe casserole dish by spraying with cooking spray.
3. Wash and scrub potatoes.
4. *Convection Cookery.* Place potatoes into a steamer and cook until tender.
   or
   Microwave Cookery. Spread potatoes over a large flat microwave-safe plate and cover with vented plastic wrap. Microwave on high for approx. 7 minutes or until potatoes are tender.
5. Place potatoes into prepared casserole dish.

6. Place chicken cubes into a large non-stick frying pan and cook over a low heat until tender. Add to potatoes in casserole dish.
7. *Convection Cookery.* Place broccoli into a steamer and cook until just tender.

    or

    Microwave Cookery. Spread broccoli over a large flat microwave-safe plate. Cover with vented plastic wrap. Microwave on high for approx. 5 minutes or until broccoli is just tender.
8. Add broccoli to potato and chicken in casserole dish.
9. Mix soy sauce, sherry and herbs and pour into casserole dish.
10. *Convection Cookery.* Bake for approx. 8 minutes or until heated through.

    or

    Microwave Cookery. Microwave on high for approx. 4 minutes or until heated through.
11. Remove cloves and bay leaves.
12. Add bean sprouts and toss lightly.

Serves 6.

CHICKEN CURRY

This is a delicious chicken curry. It has no added salt, sugar or fat. It can be made ahead of time and frozen until required. It can be served on a bed of cooked brown rice and accompanied by a salad.

INGREDIENTS
4 cups diced cooked chicken
(all skin and fat removed)
1 small onion, peeled and finely chopped
¼ cup finely chopped shallots
1 clove garlic, peeled and crushed
½ cup finely chopped green capsicum
250 g (8 ozs) firm tofu, cut into 2 cm (1″) cubes
⅓ cup natural dried raisins, cut in half
1 stick celery, finely chopped
1 apple, cored and cut into small dice
1 tablespoon curry powder (more or less, as desired)

METHOD
1. Mix all the ingredients together.
2. *Convection Cookery.* Place into a large saucepan or frying pan and heat through.
   or
   Microwave Cookery. Place into a large microwave-safe bowl. Microwave on high for approx. 8 minutes or until heated through.

Serves 4-6.

CHICKEN WITH PLUM SAUCE

This chicken recipe has a delicious plum sauce. When I make it for dinner guests it is always a great success. The chicken can be served with salad and jacket potatoes.

INGREDIENTS
1 teaspoon polyunsaturated vegetable oil
1 kg (2 lb) chicken fillets (all skin and fat removed)
2 cups stewed pitted plums (sweetened as desired)
¼ cup vinegar
2 tablespoons maize cornflour
1 cup water
2 tablespoons Sunfarm rice bran

METHOD
1. Heat oil in a large non-stick frying pan.
2. Add chicken fillets and cook until golden brown on both sides. Set aside in a large, flat oven-proof or microwave-safe dish and keep warm.
3. Add plums and vinegar to pan.
4. Place cornflour into a small bowl. Add a little water and blend well. Gradually stir in remaining water. Stir in rice bran. Add to pan and stir until mixture boils and thickens.
5. Pour sauce over chicken.
6. Reheat if desired.

Serves 6.

CHICKEN SATAY

This is a delicious way of preparing chicken. Chicken pieces are marinated overnight to develop flavour. Satay sticks are best soaked in warm water for 1 hour before they are required. Chicken Satay can be served on a bed of rice with a side salad.

INGREDIENTS

CHICKEN
500 g (1 lb) chicken fillets
  (all skin and fat removed)
12 satay sticks (soaked)

MARINADE
2 tablespoons brown sugar
1 clove garlic, peeled and crushed
½ cup soy sauce (low-salt, wheat-free)
juice of ½ lemon
1 tablespoon olive oil

SATAY SAUCE
4 tablespoons tahini
½ teaspoon paprika
⅓ cup white vinegar
3 tablespoons brown sugar
1 tablespoon olive oil
1 onion, peeled and finely chopped
1 teaspoon soy sauce (low-salt)
1 tablespoon maize cornflour
1 cup water

METHOD

CHICKEN
1. Cut chicken fillets into approx. 2 cm (1″) pieces.
2. Place chicken pieces into a large flat container with a lid.

MARINADE
1.   Mix marinade ingredients together and pour over chicken.
2.   Seal container and refrigerate overnight.
3.   Next day remove chicken pieces from marinade. Reserve marinade.
4.   Thread chicken pieces onto satay sticks.
5.   Place chicken under griller and cook, turning frequently until chicken is tender.
6.   While chicken is cooking, prepare Satay Sauce.

SATAY SAUCE
1.   Pour reserved marinade into a small bowl.
2.   Add remaining ingredients except cornflour and water.
3.   Place cornflour into a small bowl. Add a little water and blend well. Gradually stir in remaining water. Pour into sauce ingredients and stir well.
4.   *Convection Cookery.* Pour into a small saucepan. Stir over low heat until sauce boils and thickens.

or

Microwave Cookery. Pour into a small microwave-safe bowl. Microwave on high for 1 minute and stir. Continue to microwave on high stirring at 1 minute intervals until sauce boils and thickens.
5.   Pour Satay Sauce over chicken to serve.

Serves 6.

CRISPY CHICKEN PIECES

These chicken pieces are suitable to serve for a party. They have fibre added to the coating and are accompanied by a tasty sauce.

INGREDIENTS
500 g (1 lb) chicken fillets
   (all skin and fat removed)
maize cornflour for rolling chicken pieces,
   approx. ½ cup
2 egg whites, lightly beaten
Sunfarm rice bran for rolling, approx 1 cup
olive oil (for cooking)
1 tablespoon maize cornflour (extra)
1 cup apple juice (no added sugar)
1 tablespoon Worcestershire sauce
   (low-salt, wheat-free)
1 tablespoon soy sauce (low-salt, wheat-free)
1 tablespoon dry sherry

METHOD
1. Cut chicken fillets into small pieces.
2. Toss chicken pieces in cornflour. Brush with egg white. Roll in rice bran.
3. Heat a little oil in a non-stick frying pan.
4. Cook some chicken pieces until golden brown, turning frequently. Set aside in a large flat convection or microwave-safe dish and keep warm while cooking remaining chicken pieces. Add a little more oil as necessary and cook remaining chicken pieces.
5. *Convection Cookery.* Place extra cornflour into a small saucepan. Add a little apple juice and blend well. Gradually stir in remaining apple juice. Stir in sauces and sherry. Cook over a gentle heat,

stirring continuously until sauce boils and thickens.

or

Microwave Cookery. Place extra cornflour into a small microwave-safe bowl. Add a little apple juice and blend well. Gradually stir in remaining apple juice. Stir in sauces and sherry. Microwave on high for 30 seconds and stir. Continue to microwave on high stirring at 30 second intervals until sauce boils and thickens.

6. Pour sauce into a serving bowl and serve with chicken pieces.
7. Reheat chicken pieces if desired.

Makes approx. 40 chicken pieces.

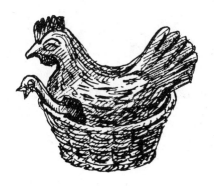

CHINESE CHICKEN

INGREDIENTS

1 x No. 16 fresh chicken
½ cup tomato sauce (low-salt)
2 tablespoons tomato paste (low-salt)
2 tablespoons soy sauce (low-salt, wheat-free)
2 tablespoons dry sherry
1 tablespoon herb or white vinegar
1 cup Taco Sauce (low-salt) (see recipe page 171)
1 clove garlic, peeled and crushed
1 x 2 cm (1") piece green ginger,
  peeled and chopped
2 tablespoons concentrated apple juice
  (no added sugar)

METHOD

1. Wash chicken and pat dry.
2. Cut into sections, taking care to remove all skin and fat.
3. Place into a flat oven-proof or microwave-safe casserole dish.
4. Blend all the remaining ingredients in the bowl of an electric food processor or blender.
5. Pour marinade over chicken.
6. Cover and place in refrigerator overnight.
7. *Convection Cookery.* Place into a cold oven. Turn oven to 180°C (350°F). Bake for approx. 1½ hours or until chicken is tender, turning once during cooking.

or

   Microwave Cookery. Microwave on high for 15 minutes. Turn chicken and microwave on medium for a further 20 minutes approx. or until chicken is tender.

Serves 6.

FISH KEBABS

This is an excellent dish to cook in the microwave oven. Care is necessary not to overcook the fish. Serve kebabs immediately on a bed of lemon and parsley rice accompanied by a tossed salad.

INGREDIENTS
500 g (1 lb) thick fish fillets (eg. gemfish or cod)
bamboo satay sticks (soaked for 1 hour)
1 punnet cherry tomatoes
1 x 425 g can baby corn (no added salt), drained and cut in half
1 stick celery, cut into 1 cm (½″) diagonal slices
2 small zucchini, cut into 1 cm (½″) diagonal slices
juice of 1 lemon
1 tablespoon polyunsaturated vegetable oil
freshly ground black pepper (as desired)

METHOD
1. Remove skin and bones from fish. Cut into 2 cm (1″) cubes.
2. Thread fish, tomatoes, corn, celery and zucchini alternately onto bamboo skewers.
3. Combine remaining ingredients and stir well. Brush glaze onto kebabs.
4. *Convection Cookery.* Place kebabs into a non-stick frying pan. Cook for approx. 5 minutes. Turn and brush again with glaze. Cook for a further 3 minutes or until cooked.
    Microwave Cookery. Preheat a microwave browning dish on high for 6 minutes. Carefully spray with cooking spray. Place kebabs onto hot dish. Microwave on high for 3 minutes. Turn and brush again with glaze. Microwave on high for a further 2 minutes or until cooked.

Serves 4.

FISH CAKES

These fish cakes are an alternative for a meat-free diet. They can be served with salad and rice.

INGREDIENTS
6 medium potatoes
300 g (10 ozs) cooked fish
½ cup Sunfarm rice bran
½ cup chopped shallots
1 teaspoon dried basil
½ teaspoon dried thyme
½ teaspoon dried oregano
cornflour for rolling fish cakes, approx. ½ cup
2 egg whites, lightly beaten, for coating
fine wholemeal breadcrumbs for coating,
    approx. 1 cup
polyunsaturated oil (for cooking)

METHOD
1. Peel potatoes and cut into small dice.
2. *Convection Cookery.* Place potato into a steamer and cook until tender.

or

   Microwave Cookery. Spread potato over a large flat microwave-safe plate. Cover with vented plastic wrap. Microwave on high for approx. 10 minutes or until potato is tender.
3. Place potato into a large bowl and mash well.
4. Flake fish and add to potato.
5. Add rice bran, shallots and herbs and mix well.
6. Shape into flat fish cakes.
7. Toss each fish cake in cornflour, egg and breadcrumbs.
8. Heat a little oil in a non-stick frying pan.

9. Place fish cakes into pan and cook until golden brown on both sides. Set aside and keep warm.
10. Add more oil as necessary and continue to cook fish cakes until all are cooked.

Makes approx. 20 fish cakes.

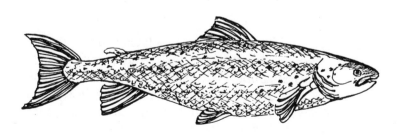

FISH LASAGNE

Most people enjoy lasagne. This recipe presents the ever popular food using fish instead of meat. You could make a meat lasagne by substituting 500 g (1 lb) of lean minced steak instead of fish.

INGREDIENTS
FISH SAUCE
2 teaspoons olive oil
650 g (1¼ lb) cooked fish fillets
1 small onion, peeled and finely chopped
2 x 475 g cans peeled tomatoes (no added salt)
125 g (4 ozs) mushrooms, sliced
1 clove garlic, peeled and crushed
1 teaspoon dried oregano
½ teaspoon dried basil
½ teaspoon dried rosemary
1 teaspoon raw sugar

LASAGNE SAUCE
2 teaspoons olive oil
2 tablespoons cornflour
2 cups soy drink
freshly ground black pepper (as desired)
¼ teaspoon nutmeg
2 cups grated tofu cheddar cheese alternative
250 g (8 ozs) wholemeal instant lasagne noodles
¼ cup soy drink (to pour over lasagne)

METHOD
FISH SAUCE
1. Heat oil in a large non-stick frying pan.
2. Flake fish fillets with a fork. Add to frying pan.
3. Add remaining Fish Sauce ingredients and cook for approx. 20 minutes over a low heat until ingredients are well combined and slightly thickened. Set aside. Prepare Lasagne Sauce.

LASAGNE SAUCE

1. *Convection Cookery.* Pour oil into a small saucepan. Stir in cornflour. Cook for 1 minute, stirring continuously. Remove from heat, add a little soy drink and blend well. Gradually stir in remaining soy drink. Stir over a low heat until sauce boils and thickens.

   or

   Microwave Cookery. Pour oil into a small microwave-safe bowl. Stir in cornflour. Add a little soy drink and blend well. Gradually stir in remaining soy drink. Microwave on high for 1 minute and stir. Continue to microwave on high, stirring at 1 minute intervals, until sauce boils and thickens.

2. Stir in black pepper, nutmeg and 1 cup grated tofu cheddar cheese alternative. Set aside.

TO FINISH

1. Preheat oven to 200°C (400°F) for convection cookery.
2. Prepare a 28 cm x 18 cm (11" x 7") flat convection or microwave-safe dish by spraying with cooking spray.
3. Line bottom of dish with lasagne noodles.
4. Spread half the Fish Sauce over the lasagne noodles.
5. Pour half the Lasagne Sauce over the Fish Sauce
6. Repeat with layers of lasagne noodles, Fish Sauce and Lasagne Sauce, finishing with noodles.
7. Pour the ¼ cup soy drink over lasagne noodles.
8. Sprinkle with remaining grated tofu cheddar cheese alternative.
9. *Convection Cookery.* Bake for approx. 20 minutes or until golden brown and heated through.

   or

   Microwave Cookery. Microwave on medium high for approx. 10 minutes or until heated through.

Serves 6-8.

FISH AND SPINACH RICE

This is an interesting way to serve fish. It is nutritious and the rice adds fibre.

INGREDIENTS
500 g (1 lb) cooked fish fillets
1 cup quick brown rice
2 cups hot water
5 spinach leaves
1 tablespoon olive oil
1 onion, peeled and finely chopped
1 clove garlic, peeled and crushed
1 teaspoon dried mixed herbs (Italian variety)
1½ cups fresh wholemeal breadcrumbs
1 tablespoon canola oil
1 tablespoon finely chopped fresh parsley

METHOD
1. Remove all skin and bones from fish fillets and flake with a fork.
2. *Convection Cookery.* Place rice and water into a large saucepan and cook until rice is tender.

   or

   Microwave Cookery. Place rice and water into a large microwave-safe bowl. Microwave on high for 5 minutes and stir. Continue to microwave on high, stirring at 1 minute intervals, until rice is tender.
3. Strain any liquid from rice.
4. Remove stalks from spinach and shred leaves. Stalks can be reserved and used as a vegetable if desired.
5. *Convection Cookery.* Place spinach leaves into a steamer and cook until just changing colour.

   or

Microwave Cookery. Place spinach leaves into a large flat microwave-safe bowl. Cover with vented plastic wrap. Microwave on high for 2 minutes and stir. Microwave on high for a further 1 minute.

6. Heat olive oil in a large non-stick frying pan. Lightly cook onion and garlic. Stir in flaked fish, spinach and rice and heat through. Place into a heat-proof serving dish and set aside to keep warm.
7. Mix herbs throughout breadcrumbs.
8. Heat canola oil in a non-stick frying pan. Add breadcrumb mixture and cook until golden brown. Stir in parsley.
9. Sprinkle breadcrumb mixture over Fish and Spinach Rice. Reheat if necessary.

Serves 6.

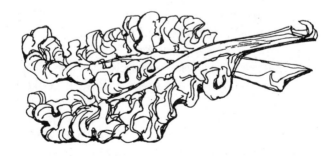

TROUT WITH ALMONDS

This recipe can be cooked in the microwave oven. The flesh is soft and moist and the almonds add a delicious flavour. Trout can be served with salad, rice or vegetables as desired.

INGREDIENTS
4 small trout, cleaned and soaked

ALMOND STUFFING
1 teaspoon canola oil
½ cup almond slivers
½ cup fine fresh wholemeal breadcrumbs
1 tablespoon soy sauce (low-salt)
1 small onion, peeled and finely chopped
2 tablespoons finely chopped shallots (for garnish)
lemon rings (for garnish)

METHOD
1. Preheat oven to 160°C (325°F) for convection cooking.
2. Wash trout and pat dry with paper towel.
3. Prepare a rectangular convection or microwave-safe dish by spraying with cooking spray.
4. Mask tail and head of trout with foil and place into prepared dish.
5. *Convection Cookery.* Bake for approx. 15 minutes or until flesh is cooked when tested.
   or
   Microwave Cookery. Microwave on defrost for approx. 12 minutes or until flesh is cooked when tested.
6. While fish is cooking prepare Almond Stuffing.
7. Place oil into a non-stick frying pan. Add almond slivers and stir over a high heat until golden brown. Reduce heat and add breadcrumbs, soy

sauce and onion. Stir continuously until onion is cooked.

8. Divide breadcrumb mixture evenly into 4 portions. Fill cavity in each trout with breadcrumb mixture. Place any remaining mixture over trout.

9. Garnish with shallots and lemon rings.

Serves 4.

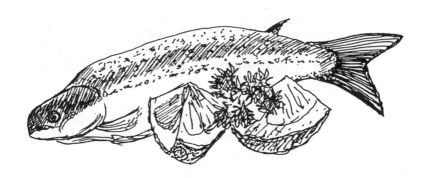

TUNA LOAF

This Tuna Loaf is ideal to serve hot with vegetables or cold with salad.

INGREDIENTS
½ cup quick brown rice
1 cup boiling water
1 x 425 g can tuna (no added salt or oil)
1 onion, peeled and cut into quarters
1 clove garlic, peeled and cut into quarters
1 carrot, peeled and roughly chopped
1 tablespoon finely chopped fresh parsley
2 tablespoons tomato paste (no added salt)
½ teaspoon dried basil
1 teaspoon concentrated vegetable stock
1 egg white

METHOD
1. Preheat oven to 180°C (350°F) for convection cooking.
2. Prepare a 23 cm x 13 cm (9" x 5") loaf tin for convection cookery or a 23 cm (9") microwave-safe ring mould by spraying with cooking spray.
3. Place rice into boiling water and cook with the lid off until rice is just tender. Strain rice and discard any remaining liquid.
4. Place tuna, onion, garlic, carrot, parsley, tomato paste, basil and stock into the bowl of an electric food processor or blender and blend until smooth.
5. Add rice and mix well.
6. In a separate, clean, dry bowl, beat egg white until stiff and lightly fold into mixture.
7. Spread into prepared tin or mould.
8. *Convection Cookery.* Bake for approx. 30 minutes or until firm.

or

Microwave Cookery. Microwave on high for approx. 6 minutes or until firm. Allow to stand for 10 minutes before turning out.

9. If loaf is to be served cold, leave in tin or mould to cool.

Serves 6-8.

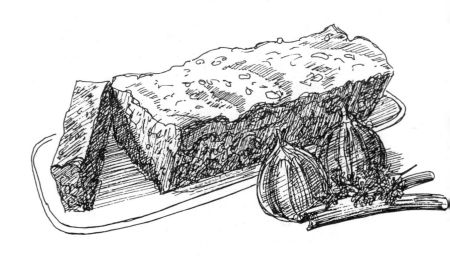

TASTY SALMON MOULD

This mould is suitable to serve as a pâté, entrée or salad accompaniment.

INGREDIENTS
500 g (1 lb) smoked salmon
1 x 250 g carton tofu pâté
1 tomato, finely diced
2 tablespoons finely chopped chives
2 tablespoons finely chopped celery
1 teaspoon finely chopped fresh basil
2 tablespoons gelatine
1 cup chicken stock

METHOD
1. Prepare a 1 litre (1½ pt) fluted mould by spraying with cooking spray.
2. Using a fork, flake salmon into a medium sized mixing bowl. Add remaining ingredients except gelatine and stock. Stir well to combine ingredients.
3. Place gelatine into a small bowl. Stir in stock. Allow to stand for 3 minutes.
4. *Convection Cookery.* Place soaked gelatine into a small saucepan. Heat gently until liquid boils.
    or
    Microwave Cookery. Place soaked gelatine into a small microwave-safe bowl. Microwave on high for 30 seconds and stir. Microwave on high for a further 20 seconds or until liquid boils.
5. Pour liquid into ingredients in bowl and stir well. Pour into prepared mould.
6. Refrigerate until firm.
7. Turn out onto a flat plate to serve.

Serves 6.

MEATBALLS

This recipe is designed to be made into small party size meat balls.

INGREDIENTS
500 g (1 lb) lean minced steak
1 tablespoon soy sauce (low-salt, wheat-free)
1 tablespoon Worcestershire sauce
  (low-salt, wheat-free)
1 teaspoon dried basil leaves
¼ teaspoon nutmeg
¼ teaspoon cumin
1 tablespoon finely chopped fresh parsley
½ teaspoon dried mixed herbs
1 clove garlic, peeled and crushed
2 tablespoons tomato paste (no added salt)
2 tablespoons Sunfarm rice bran
olive oil (for cooking)

METHOD
1. Place mince into a large mixing bowl.
2. Add remaining ingredients except olive oil and mix well.
3. Shape into small balls, approx. the size of a walnut.
4. Heat a little oil in a non-stick frying pan.
5. Cook some of the meatballs until golden brown, turning frequently. Set aside and keep warm while cooking remaining meatballs. Add a little more oil as required.

Makes approx. 40 small party meatballs.

SPAGHETTI BOLOGNESE

This recipe has no added fat or salt. It has a lovely rich tomato sauce that makes the dish good to serve to any guests. Serve with vegetables or salad.

INGREDIENTS

250 g (8 ozs) wholemeal spaghetti
4 cups boiling water
1 medium sized carrot, peeled and grated
1 medium sized zucchini, grated
½ cup chopped shallots
½ cup white wine
2 tablespoons tomato paste (no added salt)
1 x 425 g can whole peeled tomatoes
  (no added salt)
1 clove garlic, peeled and crushed
½ cup beef or vegetable stock
500 g (1 lb) lean minced steak
1 slice fresh wholemeal bread,
  made into fine breadcrumbs
½ cup grated tofu cheddar cheese alternative

METHOD

1. Preheat oven to 200°C (400°F) for convection cookery.
2. Prepare a large flat convection or microwave-safe casserole dish by spraying with cooking spray.
3. *Convection Cookery.* Place spaghetti and boiling water into a large saucepan. Cook with lid off until spaghetti is tender.

   or

   Microwave Cookery. Place spaghetti and boiling water into a large microwave-safe bowl. Cover with vented plastic. Microwave on high for approx. 5 minutes or until spaghetti is just tender.

4. Strain spaghetti and discard water.
5. Place spaghetti into prepared casserole dish. Cover and set aside.
6. Blend carrot, zucchini, shallots, wine, tomato paste, tomatoes, garlic and stock in the bowl of an electric food processor or blender.
7. *Convection Cookery.* Place blended sauce and meat into a large saucepan and cook over a gentle heat with the lid on for 20 minutes. Remove lid and cook for a further 10 minutes or until meat is cooked and sauce is thickened as desired. Stir occasionally to prevent sticking.

   or

   Microwave Cookery. Place blended sauce and meat into a large microwave-safe bowl. Microwave on medium high for approx. 10 minutes or until meat is tender. Stir occasionally during cooking.
8. Pour meat sauce over spaghetti.
9. Mix breadcrumbs and tofu cheddar cheese alternative together and sprinkle over meat sauce.
10. *Convection Cookery.* Bake for approx. 20 minutes or until heated through and breadcrumbs are golden brown.

    or

    Microwave Cookery. Microwave on high for approx. 6 minutes or until heated through. The topping will not brown unless you use a convection microwave oven.

Serves 6.

POTATO AND HAM CROQUETTES

These croquettes are suitable for a party or as an entrée.

INGREDIENTS
1 large potato
200 g (7 ozs) lean leg ham, finely chopped
3 tablespoons Sunfarm rice bran
1 tablespoon finely chopped fresh mint
½ cup finely chopped shallots
¼ teaspoon dried thyme
¼ teaspoon ground nutmeg
½ teaspoon dried sage
½ teaspoon finely chopped fresh rosemary
cornflour for rolling, approx. ½ cup
2 egg whites, lightly beaten
wheat germ for rolling, approx. 1 cup
olive oil (for cooking)

METHOD
1. Peel potato and cut into small pieces.
2. *Convection Cookery.* Place potato into a steamer and cook until soft.

   or

   Microwave Cookery. Spread potato over a large flat microwave-safe plate. Cover with vented plastic wrap. Microwave on high for approx. 6 minutes or until potato is soft.
3. Place potato into a large bowl and mash well.
4. Stir ham, rice bran and herbs into potato and mix well.
5. Shape into small cylindrical croquettes.
6. Toss croquettes in cornflour. Brush with egg white. Roll in wheat germ.
7. Heat a little oil in a non-stick frying pan.
8. Cook some of the croquettes until lightly golden

brown, turning frequently. Take care when turning croquettes. Set aside and keep warm while cooking remaining croquettes. Add a little more oil as required.

Makes approx. 20 small party size croquettes.

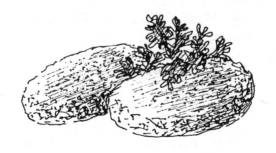

LAMB PIES

The addition of Kellogg's* All-Bran† adds fibre to the Meat Filling in this recipe.

INGREDIENTS
MEAT FILLING
500 g (1 lb) lean minced lamb
1 x 425 g can peeled tomatoes (no added salt)
½ cup Kellogg's All-Bran†*
1 tablespoon finely chopped fresh parsley
2 tablespoons tomato paste (no added salt)
1 tablespoon Worcestershire sauce (no added salt)
freshly ground black pepper (as desired)

PASTRY
2 cups wholemeal flour
1 cup wholemeal self-raising flour
*3 tablespoons polyunsaturated margarine
    (milk-free)*
¾ cup water

METHOD
MEAT FILLING
1. Place Meat Filling ingredients into a large saucepan and cook with the lid on for 20 minutes, stirring occasionally.
2. Allow Meat Filling to cool slightly while preparing pastry.

PASTRY
1. Preheat oven to 200°C (400°F).
2. Prepare 2 muffin trays by spraying with cooking spray.
3. Mix flours in a medium sized mixing bowl.
4. Rub margarine into flours until the mixture resembles fine breadcrumbs. This process may be

done by hand or with the aid of an electric food processor.

5.   Add water and mix to a firm dough.
6.   Turn dough out onto a lightly floured board and knead lightly. Roll out to 0.5 cm (¼″) thickness.
7.   Using a 10 cm (4″) round shape and a 6 cm (2½″) round shape, mark and cut out an equal number of pastry circles. (Approx. 24 of each.)
8.   Place 10 cm (4″) pastry circles into prepared muffin trays.
9.   Add a tablespoon Meat Filling to each.
10. Top each with a 6 cm (2½″) pastry circle.
11. Bake for approx. 20 minutes or until cooked when tested.
12. When cooked, remove from oven and leave in trays for 15 minutes before turning out onto a fine wire rack to cool.

Makes approx. 24 pies.

LAMB AND VEGETABLE PIE

The combination of lamb and vegetables makes this a very tasty pie. The addition of Kellogg's* All-Bran† adds fibre to the pie. This pie can be served hot or cold as desired.

INGREDIENTS

LAMB AND VEGETABLE FILLING
3 ripe tomatoes
500 g (1 lb) lean minced lamb
1 carrot, peeled and coarsely grated
1 small zucchini, coarsely grated
2 stalks celery, finely chopped
¼ cup finely chopped shallots
1 tablespoon finely chopped fresh parsley
1 teaspoon dried oregano
½ teaspoon dried dill tips
¼ teaspoon dried mixed herbs
freshly ground black pepper (as desired)
2 tablespoons tomato paste (no added salt)
1 cup Kellogg's All-Bran†*

PASTRY
2 cups wholemeal flour
1 cup wholemeal self-raising flour
*3 tablespoons polyunsaturated margarine
    (milk-free)*
¾ cup water

METHOD

LAMB AND VEGETABLE FILLING
1. Place tomatoes into boiling water and leave for 1 minute. Remove skins and cut tomatoes into small dice.
2. Place Lamb and Vegetable Filling ingredients into a large saucepan and cook with the lid on over a gentle heat for 15 minutes, stirring occasionally.

3. Allow to cool while preparing Pastry.

PASTRY
1. Preheat oven to 200°C (400°F).
2. Prepare a 28 cm x 20 cm (11″ x 8″) deep pie dish by spraying with cooking spray.
3. Mix flours in a medium sized mixing bowl.
4. Rub margarine into flours until the mixture resembles fine breadcrumbs. This process may be done by hand or with the aid of an electric food processor.
5. Add water and mix to a firm dough.
6. Turn dough out onto a lightly floured board and knead lightly. Roll out two-thirds to approx. 0.5 cm (¼″) thickness to fit base and sides of pie dish.
7. Line prepared dish with pastry.
8. Place Lamb and Vegetable Filling onto pastry.
9. Roll out remaining pastry and cover filling. Press edges of pastry together.
10. Bake for approx. 40 minutes or until cooked when tested.

Serves 8-10.

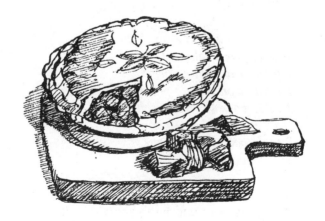

PORK AND LAMB SURPRISE

This is a delicious combination of lean pork and lamb with the addition of peaches to add to its appeal. If you are in a hurry it isn't necessary to marinate the meat, however it does give the finished dish more flavour. The Pork and Lamb Surprise may be served in the wok if you like, to save using another dish, or it can be placed into a large casserole dish.

INGREDIENTS
PORK AND LAMB SURPRISE
500 g (1 lb) lean pork short cuts
500 g (1 lb) lean lamb short cuts
½ cup maize cornflour
1 x 425 g can peach slices in natural juice
2 tablespoons soy sauce (low-salt, wheat-free)
1 clove garlic, peeled and crushed
1 tablespoon soya bean oil
½ cup finely chopped shallots
½ cup thin red capsicum strips
½ cup thin green capsicum strips
1 cup thin celery strips
1 ripe banana

WINE SAUCE
3 tablespoons maize cornflour
3 tablespoons cold water
1 tablespoon white vinegar
1 tablespoon tomato paste (no added salt)
1 tablespoon Worcestershire sauce
   (low-salt, wheat-free)
1 tablespoon brown sugar
½ cup white wine

METHOD
1.   Toss pork and lamb short cuts in cornflour.

2. Place meat into a large container with a lid.
3. Strain juice from peaches into a small bowl. Place peach slices in a covered container and refrigerate. These are to be kept to decorate the finished dish just before serving.
4. Stir soy sauce and garlic into peach juice. Pour over meat.
5. Cover and marinate in the refrigerator overnight.
6. Next day, place oil into a large wok or electric frypan.
7. Heat oil at approx. 7 on a dial of 1-10.
8. Add marinated meat.
9. Stir fry for approx. 10 minutes or until meat is tender.
10. Add shallots, capsicum and celery strips and stir-fry for 2 minutes.
11. Peel banana and cut into small dice. Stir into wok. Turn wok off while preparing Wine Sauce

WINE SAUCE
1. Place cornflour into a small bowl. Add a little water and blend well. Gradually stir in remaining water. Stir in remaining ingredients and mix well.
2. *Convection Cookery.* Pour sauce into a small saucepan. Stir over a low heat until sauce boils and thickens.

or

   Microwave Cookery. Pour sauce into a small microwave-safe bowl. Microwave on high for 1 minute and stir. Continue to microwave on high, stirring at 1 minute intervals until sauce boils and thickens.
3. Turn wok on again and pour in Wine Sauce. Stir for 1 minute.
4. To serve in wok or casserole dish, arrange peach slices around the outer edge of the meat. They add nutrition to the dish, as well as flavour and colour.

Serves 6.

OSSO BUCCO

This is a traditional Italian dish you can prepare in a low-fat form. This tasty dish is easy to prepare and will delight your palate. It has no added fat or salt. It is possible to partly cook this casserole in the convection oven and finish it in the microwave to save time.

INGREDIENTS
OSSO BUCCO
2 lean veal shanks, cut into approx. 4 pieces each
¼ cup maize cornflour
1 large carrot, peeled and cut into small dice
2 sticks celery, cut into small dice
2 onions, peeled and cut into small dice
1 x 425 g can peeled tomatoes (no added salt)
1 cup dry white wine
1 teaspoon dried basil
1 teaspoon dried lemon balm
1 bay leaf

GREMOLADA
finely grated rind of 1 lemon
2 cloves garlic, peeled and crushed
2 tablespoons finely chopped fresh parsley

METHOD
OSSO BUCCO
1. Prepare a large convection or microwave-safe casserole dish with lid by spraying with cooking spray.
2. Trim any visible fat from veal shanks.
3. Toss veal shanks in cornflour. Place into prepared casserole dish. Sprinkle any remaining cornflour over veal shanks.
4. Place carrot, celery and onion over meat.
5. Mix tomatoes, wine, basil and lemon balm

together. Pour over meat and vegetables. Add bay leaf.
6. Cover and marinate in the refrigerator overnight.
7. *Convection Cookery.* Next day, place covered into a cold oven. Turn oven to 180°C (350°F) and bake for approx. 1½ hours or until meat is tender.
or
Microwave Cookery. Next day, microwave, covered, on high for 10 minutes then microwave on defrost for approx. 1½ hours, stirring occasionally until meat is tender.
8. Prepare Gremolada.

GREMOLADA
1. Combine ingredients and stir into Osso Bucco.
2. *Convection Cookery.* Bake uncovered for 10 minutes.
or
Microwave Cookery. Cover with vented plastic and microwave on high for 5 minutes.

Serves 6-8 depending on the size of the veal shanks.

VEAL IN RED WINE

INGREDIENTS
500 g (1 lb) lean veal slices
2 tablespoons potato flour
1 large onion, peeled and finely chopped
2 cloves garlic, peeled and crushed
500 g (1 lb) potatoes, peeled and cut into small cubes
1 large carrot, peeled and cut into small cubes
1 stick celery, finely chopped
1 cup red wine
2 tablespoons tomato paste (no added salt)
2 cups stock
2 tablespoons soy sauce (low-salt, wheat-free)
¼ teaspoon each of dried basil, sage, marjoram, thyme
freshly ground black pepper (as desired)
2 bay leaves
6 whole cloves
12 prunes, pitted
12 dried apricot halves

METHOD
1. Preheat oven to 180°C (350°F).
2. Prepare a large casserole dish with lid by spraying with cooking spray.
3. Toss veal slices in potato flour.
4. Place veal slices into prepared casserole dish.
5. Add onion, garlic, potato, carrot and celery to casserole dish.
6. In a medium sized mixing bowl, combine red wine, tomato paste, stock, soy sauce, herbs and pepper. Pour into casserole dish.
7. Add bay leaves, cloves, prunes and apricots.
8. Cover and cook for approx. 45 minutes or until veal and vegetables are tender.
9. Remove bay leaves and cloves before serving.

Serves 6.

VEAL AND VEGETABLE LOAF

A combination of lean minced veal and vegetables makes this a tasty meat loaf. Each loaf will serve 6 according to recommended daily meat allowances. It can be served hot with vegetables or cold with salad. If you require only one loaf immediately, the other will freeze well for later use.

INGREDIENTS
1 kg (2 lb) lean minced veal
1 large carrot, peeled and finely grated
1 small zucchini, finely grated
2 cups Sweet and Sour Sauce (see recipe page 173)
1 cup firm tofu, cut into small cubes
½ cup tomato paste (no added salt)
1 teaspoon dried mixed herbs (French variety)
1 egg white, lightly beaten

METHOD
1. Preheat oven to 150°C (300°F).
2. Prepare two 23 cm x 13 cm (9" x 5") loaf tins by spraying with cooking spray.
3. Combine all the ingredients and mix well.
4. Press into prepared loaf tins.
5. Bake for approx. 45 minutes or until cooked as desired.
6. Serve hot or cold as desired.

BEANS BORLOTTI

Borlotti beans are a favourite in Italian and Middle Eastern cookery. The beans have a smooth texture and a nutty flavour. They readily absorb other flavours and make an ideal high-fibre addition for this recipe.

INGREDIENTS
200 g (7 ozs) borlotti beans
3 cups boiling water
2 medium sized onions, peeled and finely chopped
2 sticks celery, finely chopped
½ red capsicum, seeded and finely chopped
½ green capsicum, seeded and finely chopped
1 large carrot, peeled and finely grated
1 small-medium zucchini, grated
1 teaspoon freshly crushed garlic
¼ teaspoon dried dill tips
½ teaspoon dried salad herbs
½ teaspoon dried mixed herbs
¼ teaspoon dried rosemary
¼ teaspoon dried tarragon
¼ teaspoon dried thyme
2 tablespoons maize cornflour
1 cup water
1 teaspoon concentrated vegetable stock
1 tablespoon soy sauce (low-salt, wheat-free)
1 tablespoon Worcestershire sauce
    (low-salt, wheat-free)

METHOD
1. Place beans and boiling water into a large saucepan. Bring to the boil, uncovered. Reduce heat and simmer for 5 minutes.
2. Place lid on saucepan and allow to stand for 1 hour.

3. Strain beans and discard liquid.
4. Preheat oven to 180°C (350°F) for convection cookery.
5. Prepare a 2 litre (3 pt) convection or microwave-safe casserole dish .by spraying with cooking spray.
6. Place beans into prepared dish.
7. Add vegetables and herbs and mix well.
8. *Convection Cookery.* Place cornflour into a small saucepan. Add a little water and blend well. Gradually stir in remaining water. Add vegetable stock and sauces. Cook over a low heat, stirring continuously until sauce boils and thickens.

or

Microwave Cookery. Place cornflour into a small microwave-safe bowl. Add a little water and blend well. Gradually stir in remaining water. Add vegetable stock and sauces. Microwave on high for 1 minute and stir. Continue to microwave on high, stirring at 1 minute intervals until sauce boils and thickens.
9. Pour sauce into casserole dish.
10. *Convection Cookery.* Bake for approx. 20 minutes or until heated through.

or

Microwave cookery. Microwave on high for approx. 8 minutes or until heated through, stirring occasionally.

Serves 4-6.

BEAN CASSEROLE

This casserole is made using a variety of beans. Beans add excellent fibre to the diet.

INGREDIENTS
3 large tomatoes
1 tablespoon olive oil
1 onion, peeled and chopped
1 clove garlic, peeled and crushed
¼ cup tomato paste (no added salt)
1 red capsicum, seeded and chopped
¼ cup finely chopped fresh parsley
¼ cup finely chopped fresh basil
1 x 440 g can 3 bean mix
1 x 440 g can soya beans
1 cup finely sliced fresh beans
200 g (7 ozs) mushrooms, finely sliced

METHOD
1. Preheat oven to 200°C (400°F) for convection cookery.
2. Place tomatoes into boiling water for 1 minute. Remove skins and cut into small cubes.
3. Prepare a 2 litre (3 pt) convection or microwave-safe casserole dish by spraying with cooking spray.
4. Heat oil in a non-stick frying pan. Cook onion and garlic until onion is soft. Place into prepared casserole dish.
5. Add tomato and remaining ingredients except mushrooms to casserole dish and mix well.
6. *Convection Cookery.* Bake for approx. 15 minutes or until heated through. Add mushrooms and cook for a further 3 minutes.

or

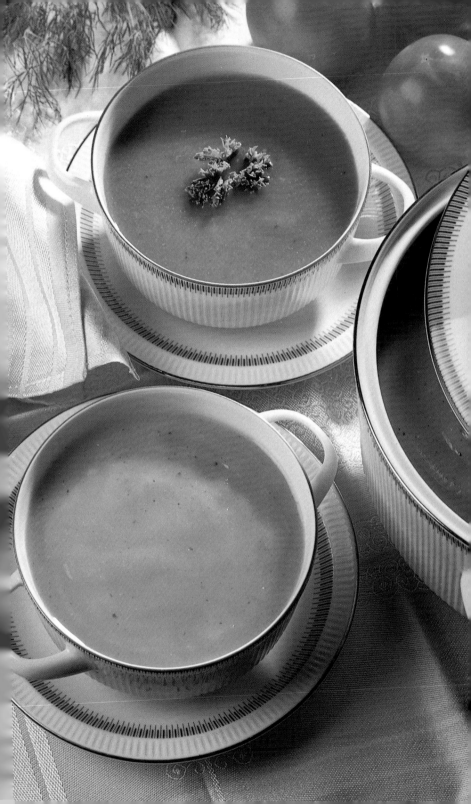

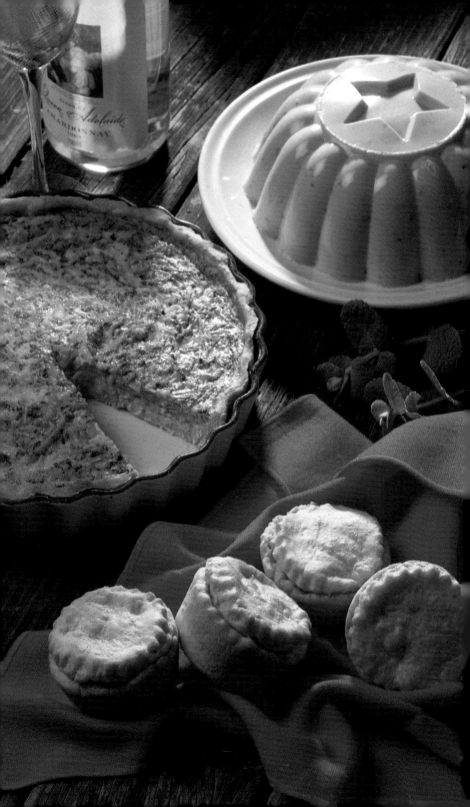

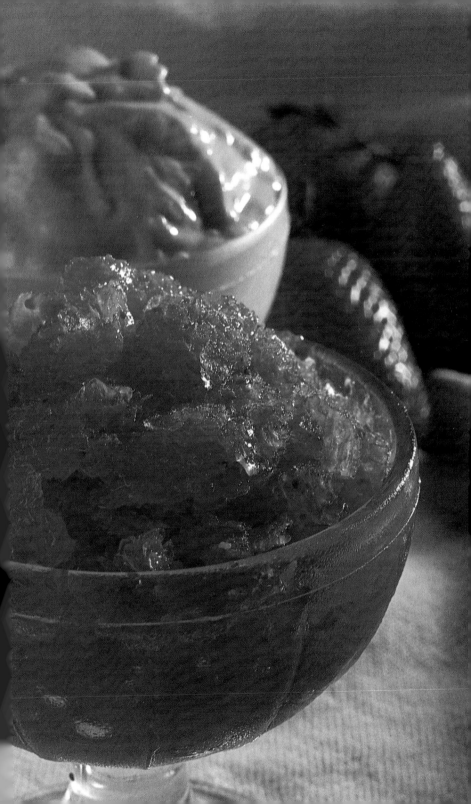

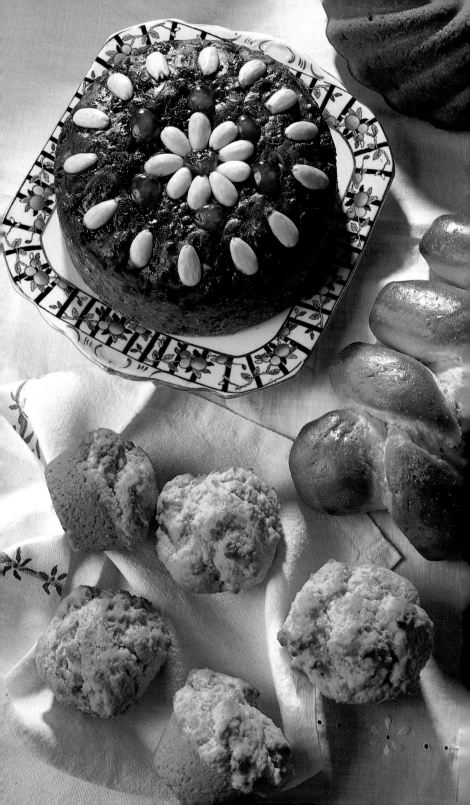

Microwave Cookery. Microwave on high for approx. 5 minutes or until heated through. Stir occasionally during cooking. Add mushrooms and microwave for a further 2 minutes.

Serves 6.

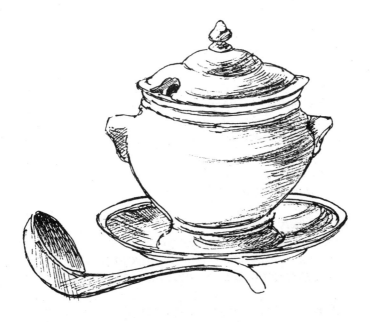

Opposite: Banana Cake (page 147), Wholemeal Bread (page 142) and Apple & Oat Bran Muffins (page 161)
Overleaf (left): Tasty Salmon Mould (page 70), Carrot Quiche (page 92) and Lamb Pies (page 76)
Overleaf (right): Tofu Ice-cream (page 130) with Tofu-Banana Cream (page 174) and Strawberry Sorbet (page 125)
Opposite page 88: Tomato Soup (page 43) and Pumpkin Vichyssoise (page 42)

BUTTERNUT RICE

Fried rice is always a popular accompaniment to a meal. This recipe has the added colour and flavour of sweet butternut pumpkin.

INGREDIENTS
1½ cups quick brown rice
1½ cups water
½ small butternut pumpkin
1 teaspoon polyunsaturated oil
⅓ cup almond slivers
½ cup chopped green capsicum
½ cup chopped red capsicum
1 cup finely chopped broccoli
1 cup corn kernels
½ cup finely chopped shallots
1 tablespoon finely chopped fresh parsley
2 tablespoons soy sauce (low-salt, wheat-free)
2 tablespoons black bean sauce (low-salt)

METHOD
1. *Convection Cookery.* Place rice and water into a large saucepan. Cook until water is absorbed and rice is tender, adding a little more water if necessary.

    or

    Microwave Cookery. Place rice and water into a large microwave-safe bowl. Cover with vented plastic wrap and cook for approx. 10 minutes or until water is absorbed and rice is tender, adding a little more water if necessary.
2. Peel and cut pumpkin into small, thin, flat strips.
3. *Convection Cookery.* Place pumpkin into a steamer and cook until just tender. Do not overcook or pumpkin will break up.

Microwave Cookery. Spread pumpkin over a large flat microwave-safe plate. Cover with vented plastic wrap. Microwave on high for approx. 5 minutes or until pumpkin is just tender.

4. Heat oil in a wok or large non-stick frying pan.
5. Add almonds and stir until golden brown.
6. Add rice, pumpkin and remaining ingredients and stir until vegetables are just tender.

Serves 4 as a main meal or 6-8 as an accompaniment to a main meal.

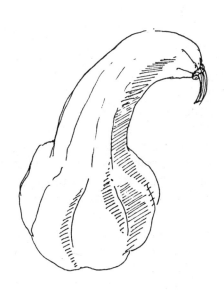

CARROT QUICHE

This quiche may be served hot or cold as desired.

INGREDIENTS
PASTRY
1 tablespoon polyunsaturated margarine (milk-free)
1 cup wholemeal self-raising flour
½ cup Kellogg's* All-Bran†
½ cup soy drink

QUICHE FILLING
1 cup finely grated carrot
1 cup soy drink
2 eggs, lightly beaten
freshly ground black pepper (as desired)
1 tablespoon finely chopped fresh parsley
¼ cup finely chopped shallots
¼ teaspoon nutmeg
½ teaspoon dried dill tips
¼ teaspoon dried sage
1 cup grated tofu cheddar cheese alternative
1 egg white

METHOD
PASTRY
1. Preheat oven to 200°C (400°F).
2. Prepare a 23 cm (9″) quiche dish by spraying with cooking spray.
3. Rub margarine into flour until mixture resembles fine breadcrumbs. This process may be done by hand or with the aid of an electric food processor.
4. Stir in All-Bran.
5. Pour ½ cup soy drink into dry ingredients and mix to a firm dough.
6. Turn dough out onto a lightly floured board and knead lightly. Roll out to 0.5 cm (¼″) thickness

to fit base and sides of prepared dish.
7.   Carefully line quiche dish with pastry.
8.   Prepare Quiche Filling.

QUICHE FILLING
1.   Mix ingredients, except egg white, together in a medium sized bowl.
2.   In a separate, clean, dry bowl, beat egg white until stiff and lightly fold into Quiche Filling.
3.   Pour Quiche Filling into prepared pastry shell.
4.   Bake for approx. 30 minutes or until set in the centre when tested.

Serves 6.

NUT LOAF

Canned nut-meat is used to make this Nut Loaf. There are a few variations of nut-meat that can be purchased which are suitable for this recipe. Nut-meats are usually milk-free, however it is important to be ever mindful of the need to read all labels before purchasing.

INGREDIENTS

1 x 430 g can nut-meat, mashed
2 medium sized carrots, peeled and grated
1 onion, peeled and grated
1 cup tomato paste (no added salt)
1 egg, well beaten
1 teaspoon dried mixed herbs (Italian variety)
1 cup grated tofu cheddar cheese alternative

METHOD

1. Preheat oven to 180°C (350°F) for convection cookery.
2. Prepare a 23 cm x 9 cm (9" x 3½") loaf tin or 23 cm (9") microwave-safe ring mould by spraying with cooking spray.
3. Place all the ingredients into a large bowl and mix well.
4. Spread into prepared tin or mould.
5. *Convection Cookery.* Bake for approx. 35 minutes or until golden brown and cooked when tested.

   or

   Microwave Cookery. Microwave on high for approx. 8 minutes or until cooked when tested.
6. When cooked, remove from oven and leave in tin or mould for 10 minutes before turning out to serve.

Serves 8.

PITA PIZZAS

These delicious pizzas contain no added fat, sugar or salt. Be sure to select milk-free pita breads.

INGREDIENTS
4 small wholemeal pita breads
4 tablespoons tomato paste (no added salt)
4 tablespoons Maria's Marvellous Taco Sauce
 (see recipe page 171)
1 large tomato
4 tablespoons finely chopped shallots
1 stalk celery, finely sliced
1 tablespoon finely chopped fresh parsley
1 cup grated tofu cheddar cheese alternative

METHOD
1. Preheat convection oven to 200°C (400°F).
2. Prepare a large flat oven tray by spraying with cooking spray.
3. Place pita breads onto prepared tray.
4. Spread evenly with tomato paste and then Taco Sauce.
5. Place tomato into boiling water for 1 minute. Remove skin and cut into thin slices and place onto pita breads.
6. Sprinkle shallot, celery and parsley evenly over pita breads.
7. Sprinkle tofu cheddar cheese alternative evenly over pita breads.
8. *Convection Cookery.* Bake for approx. 15 minutes or until golden brown.
    or
    Microwave Cookery. Microwave on high for approx. 5 minutes or until heated through.

Serves 4.

POTATO AND CELERY PIE

Vegetable pies are delicious served with salads. This pie may be served hot or cold as desired.

INGREDIENTS
PASTRY
1 tablespoon polyunsaturated margarine (milk-free)
1 cup wholemeal self-raising flour
½ cup Kellogg's* All-Bran†
½ cup soy drink

FILLING
3 medium potatoes, peeled and cut into
   1 cm (½″) cubes
1 onion, peeled and cut into 1 cm (½″) cubes
½ cup chopped celery
2 eggs, lightly beaten
1 tablespoon finely chopped fresh parsley
½ teaspoon dried sage
freshly ground black pepper (as desired)
1 cup soy drink
2 egg whites

METHOD
PASTRY
1. Preheat oven to 200°C (400°F).
2. Prepare a 23 cm (9″) pie dish by spraying with cooking spray.
3. Rub margarine into flour until mixture resembles fine breadcrumbs. This process may be done by hand or with the aid of an electric food processor.
4. Stir in All-Bran.
5. Pour soy drink into dry ingredients and mix to a firm dough.
6. Turn dough out onto a lightly floured board and knead lightly. Roll out to 0.5 cm (¼″) thickness

to fit base and sides of prepared dish.

7. Carefully line dish with pastry.
8. Prepare Filling

FILLING

1. *Convection Cookery.* Place potato, onion and celery into a steamer and cook until potato is just tender.

    or

    Microwave Cookery. Spread potato, onion and celery over a large flat microwave-safe plate. Cover with vented plastic wrap. Microwave on high for approx. 8 minutes or until potato is tender.
2. Place cooked vegetables into a medium sized mixing bowl.
3. Stir in lightly beaten eggs, herbs, pepper and soy drink.
4. In a separate, clean, dry bowl, beat egg whites until stiff and lightly fold into mixture.
5. Pour mixture into prepared pastry case.
6. Bake for approx. 30 minutes or until set in the centre when tested.

Serves 6.

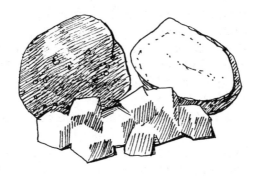

SOYA BEAN PIZZA

This recipe is designed for those who enjoy a vegetarian style pizza.

INGREDIENTS

PIZZA BASE
2 cups wholemeal flour
½ teaspoon baking powder
3 tablespoons canola oil
3 tablespoons water
1 teaspoon lemon juice

PIZZA TOPPING
4 tablespoons tomato paste (no added salt)
1 cup soya beans in tomato sauce
1 small zucchini, finely grated
1 red capsicum, seeded and cut into thin strips
100 g (3½ ozs) mushrooms, thinly sliced
1 large onion, peeled and cut into thin slices
¼ cup chopped black olives
1 teaspoon finely chopped fresh basil
1 teaspoon dried mixed herbs (Italian variety)
1 cup grated tofu cheddar cheese alternative

METHOD

PIZZA BASE
1. Preheat oven to 220°C (425°F).
2. Prepare a 30 cm (12″) pizza tray by spraying with cooking spray.
3. Place flour into a medium sized mixing bowl. Stir in baking powder.
4. Mix oil, water and lemon juice in a small jug and pour into flour. Mix well to form a firm dough. This process may be done by hand or with the aid of an electric food processor.
5. Turn dough out onto a lightly floured board and

knead lightly. Roll out to approx. 0.5 cm (¼")
thickness to fit base of prepared tray. Carefully
place onto prepared tray.

6.   Cover base with Pizza Topping.

PIZZA TOPPING

1.   Place Topping ingredients onto pastry base in
      listed order.

2.   Place pizza into oven and bake for approx. 20
      minutes or until golden brown and pastry is
      cooked.

Serves 6.

SOYA PATTIES

These nutritious patties are made with soya beans and vegetables. Dried soya beans require soaking overnight.

INGREDIENTS
½ cup dried soya beans
1 cup water
1 cup cooked mashed potato
1 small zucchini, finely grated
1 small carrot, peeled and finely grated
1 onion, peeled and finely chopped
1 tablespoon finely chopped fresh parsley
2 tablespoons tomato relish (low-salt)
1 clove garlic, peeled and crushed
1 egg, lightly beaten
1 teaspoon dried mixed herbs (Italian variety)
¼ teaspoon dried coriander
¼ teaspoon dried cumin
¼ teaspoon dried sage
maize cornflour for rolling patties, approx. ⅓ cup
olive oil (for cooking)

METHOD
1.   Soak soya beans in water overnight
2.   Next day drain beans and discard water.
3.   Blend soya beans in the bowl of an electric food processor or blender.
4.   Mix soya beans with remaining ingredients, except olive oil and cornflour.
5.   Shape mixture into patties and roll in cornflour.
6.   Heat a little oil in a non-stick frying pan. Cook patties on both sides until lightly golden brown. Take care when turning patties over.

Makes approx. 10 patties.

VEGETABLE-MANGO PATTIES

INGREDIENTS
1 x 440 g can corn kernels
2 small zucchini, grated
2 small carrots, peeled and grated
2 small onions, peeled and finely chopped
½ red capsicum, seeded and finely chopped
1 egg, lightly beaten
¼ cup polenta
¼ cup wholemeal self-raising flour
cornflour, approx. ½ cup (for rolling)
olive oil (for cooking)
1 cup fresh mango pulp ⎫
1 tablespoon white vinegar ⎬ *for mango sauce*
1 tablespoon sweet white wine ⎭

METHOD
1. Place vegetables, egg, polenta and flour into a medium sized mixing bowl and mix well.
2. Shape into flat patties. Toss patties in cornflour.
3. Heat a little oil in a non-stick frying pan.
4. Add patties and cook, turning frequently until golden brown.
5. Remove patties from pan. Set aside and keep warm while preparing sauce.
6. *Convection Cookery.* Place mango pulp, vinegar and wine into pan. Stir over a gentle heat until sauce boils.
or
   Microwave Cookery. Place mango pulp, vinegar and wine into a small microwave-safe bowl. Microwave on high for 1 minute and stir. Continue to microwave on high, stirring at 30 second intervals until sauce boils.
7. Serve sauce in a gravy bowl or over patties.

Makes approx. 6-8 patties.

WHOLEMEAL PATTIES

These patties are made from wholemeal bread and vegetables. They can be served as an accompaniment to a main meal or as a mini meal. The mixture can also be used as a stuffing for chicken. Take care when purchasing bread to ensure a milk-free product.

INGREDIENTS
2 cups fresh wholemeal breadcrumbs
1 onion, peeled and finely chopped
1 clove garlic, peeled and crushed
1 tablespoon finely chopped fresh parsley
¼ cup finely chopped celery
½ cup pine nuts
½ cup pumpkin seed kernels
½ cup mashed tofu
½ teaspoon dried mixed herbs
1 egg, lightly beaten
olive oil (for cooking)

METHOD
1. Mix all the ingredients except oil together in a large bowl.
2. Shape mixture into patties.
3. Heat a little oil in a non-stick frying pan. Cook patties on both sides until lightly golden brown. Take care when turning patties over.

Makes approx. 8 patties.

VEGETABLES AND SALADS

	MILK-FREE	WHEAT-FREE	EGG-FREE	LOW-FAT	LOW-SUGAR	CONVECTION	MICROWAVE	FREEZER
VEGETABLES								
Garlic Zucchini	•	•	•	•	•	•	•	
Ginger-Marmalade Potatoes	•	•	•	•	•	•	•	•
Honey-Ginger Carrots	•	•	•	•	•	•	•	
Potato Skins	•	•	•	•	•	•	•	
Soya-Cottage Potatoes	•	•			•	•	•	•
Tofu Potatoes	•	•	•		•	•	•	•
SALADS								
Brown Rice Salad	•	•	•	•	•	•	•	
Cauliflower Salad	•	•	•	•	•	•		
Hot Bean Salad	•	•	•	•	•	•	•	
Hot Potato Salad	•	•	•	•	•	•	•	
Waldorf-Chicken Salad	•	•	•	•	•	•	•	
Zucchini Salad	•	•	•	•	•			

GARLIC ZUCCHINI

It is important not to over-cook the zucchini to retain flavour and crispness for this delicious recipe.

INGREDIENTS
6 small-medium sized zucchini
1 teaspoon freshly crushed garlic
1 teaspoon dried salad herbs
½ teaspoon finely chopped fresh mint

METHOD
1. Cut zucchini into small cubes.
2. *Convection Cookery.* Place zucchini into a steamer and cook until just tender.

    or

    Microwave Cookery. Place zucchini into a flat microwave-safe dish. Cover with vented plastic wrap and microwave on high for approx. 4 minutes or until zucchini is just tender.
3. Place zucchini into a serving dish.
4. Add garlic and herbs and lightly toss.

Serves 6.

GINGER-MARMALADE POTATOES

INGREDIENTS

1 kg (2 lb) potatoes, peeled and cut into 1 cm (½") slices
2 tablespoons marmalade
2 tablespoons chopped green ginger
1 tablespoon herb or white vinegar
2 tablespoons honey
finely grated rind and juice of 1 orange
2 tablespoons cream sherry

METHOD

1. Preheat convection oven to 220°C (425°F).
2. Prepare a 4 litre (6 pt) flat convection or microwave-safe casserole dish by spraying with cooking spray.
3. *Convection Cookery.* Place potato slices into a steamer and cook until potato is just tender.
    Microwave Cookery. Spread potato slices over a large flat microwave-safe plate. Cover with vented plastic wrap. Microwave on high for approx. 10 minutes or until potato is just tender.
4. Arrange half the potato slices over base of prepared dish. Set remaining potato aside.
5. *Convection Cookery.* Place remaining ingredients into a small saucepan and stir well. Bring to the boil and simmer for 2 minutes.
    Microwave Cookery. Place remaining ingredients into a small microwave-safe bowl and stir well. Microwave on high for 1 minute or until boils.
6. Pour sauce over potato slices in casserole dish.
7. Arrange remaining potato slices in dish.
8. *Convection Cookery.* Bake for approx. 10 minutes or until heated through.
    Microwave Cookery. Microwave on high for approx. 5 minutes or until heated through.

Serves 10 as a side dish or 6 as a meat-alternative dish.

HONEY-GINGER CARROTS

Ginger and honey add flavour to carrots.

INGREDIENTS
3 large carrots, peeled and cut into small cubes
2 teaspoons chopped green ginger
1 tablespoon honey

METHOD
1. *Convection Cookery.* Place carrot into a steamer and cook for approx. 7 minutes or until carrot is just tender.
                          or
    Microwave Cookery. Spread carrot over a large flat microwave-safe plate. Cover with vented plastic wrap. Microwave on high for approx. 5 minutes or until carrot is just tender.
2. Place carrot into a serving bowl.
3. Add ginger and honey and toss lightly.

Serves 6.

POTATO SKINS

Potato Skins can be eaten as desired. This recipe is designed as a nibble food, dipped in sauce before eating.

INGREDIENTS
6 medium sized potatoes
¼ cup soy sauce (low-salt, wheat-free)
¼ cup lemon juice
¼ cup honey
1 clove garlic, peeled and crushed
1 teaspoon finely chopped green ginger
2 tablespoons sherry
1 tablespoon maize cornflour
1 tablespoon water

METHOD
1. Preheat oven to 200°C (400°F).
2. Scrub potatoes and towel dry.
3. Bake for approx. 55 minutes or until soft.
4. Cut into quarters and scoop out cooked potato, leaving 0.5 cm (¼") thickness. Cooked potato can be reserved and used in a casserole or soup as desired.
5. Place skins on a rack and return to oven to bake for a further 15 minutes.
6. Place remaining ingredients into a small bowl and mix well.
7. *Convection Cookery.* Place sauce into a small saucepan. Stir over a low heat until sauce boils and thickens.

or

Microwave Cookery. Place sauce into a small microwave-safe bowl. Microwave on high for 1 minute and stir. Microwave on high for a further 1 minute or until sauce boils and thickens.
8. Serve sauce in a sauce bowl.

SOYA-COTTAGE POTATOES

This recipe is a nice variation for presenting potatoes as a main meal.

INGREDIENTS

6 large potatoes, peeled and cut into small dice
500 g (1 lb) soya cottage cheese
½ cup finely chopped shallots
1 teaspoon curry powder (as desired)
2 egg whites
⅓ cup Sunfarm rice bran
½ cup grated tofu cheddar cheese alternative
1 tablespoon cashew or almond spread

METHOD

1. Preheat oven to 200°C (400°F) for convection cookery.
2. Prepare a 2 litre (3 pt) flat convection or microwave-safe casserole dish by spraying with cooking spray.
3. *Convection Cookery.* Place potato into a steamer and cook until soft.

    or

    Microwave Cookery. Spread potato over a large flat microwave-safe plate. Cover with vented plastic wrap. Microwave on high for approx. 10 minutes or until potato is soft.
4. Place potato into a large bowl and mash well.
5. Add soya cottage cheese, shallots and curry powder and mix well.
6. In a separate, clean, dry bowl, beat egg whites until stiff and lightly fold into potato mixture.
7. Spread potato mixture into prepared casserole dish.
8. Top with rice bran, tofu cheese and small dobs

of cashew or almond spread.

9. *Convection Cookery.* Bake for approx. 20 minutes or until golden brown and heated through.

or

Microwave Cookery. Microwave on high for approx. 7 minutes or until heated through.

Serves 6.

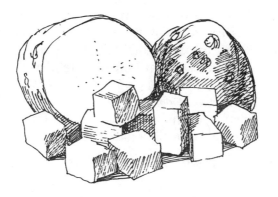

TOFU POTATOES

This recipe makes a large dish of potato suitable to serve as a side dish or as a meat-substitute meal.

INGREDIENTS
1 kg (2 lb) potatoes, peeled and cut
into 1 cm (½″) slices
1 clove garlic, peeled and crushed
freshly ground black pepper (as desired)
375 g (12 ozs) firm tofu,
cut into 0.5 cm (¼″) slices
1 litre (32 fl ozs) soy drink

METHOD
1. Preheat oven to 200°C (400°F) for convection cookery.
2. Prepare a 4 litre (6 pt) flat convection or microwave-safe casserole dish by spraying with cooking spray.
3. Arrange half the potato slices over base of prepared dish.
4. Sprinkle with crushed garlic and pepper.
5. Arrange tofu slices over potato.
6. Arrange remaining potato slices over tofu.
7. Pour soy drink over potato slices.
8. *Convection Cookery.* Cover with foil and bake for 20 minutes. Remove foil and bake for a further 20 minutes or until potato is tender.
   or
   Microwave Cookery. Cover with vented plastic wrap and microwave on high for approx. 20 minutes or until potato is tender.

Serves 12 as a side dish or 6 as a main meal.

BROWN RICE SALAD

Brown rice is high in fibre and has a firm texture. Mixed with fresh crisp vegetables, it makes a nutritious salad. This salad may be served warm or cold as desired.

INGREDIENTS
1 cup quick brown rice
1½ cups water
1 stick celery, finely chopped
1 medium carrot, peeled and grated
1 small zucchini, grated
½ red capsicum, seeded and finely chopped
½ green capsicum, seeded and finely chopped
1 tablespoon finely chopped fresh parsley

METHOD
1. *Convection Cookery.* Place rice and water into a large saucepan. Cook with lid off until rice is tender.

   or

   Microwave Cookery. Place rice and water into a large microwave-safe bowl. Microwave on high for approx. 12 minutes or until rice is tender.
2. Strain any remaining liquid from rice and place rice into a serving dish.
3. Add vegetables to rice and toss lightly.

Serves 4.

CAULIFLOWER SALAD

Fresh, crisp vegetables are excellent for this nutritious salad. Natural sultanas add a fruity flavour.

INGREDIENTS
1 small cauliflower, cut into small pieces
2 carrots, peeled and cut into thin strips
½ cup chopped chives
1 red capsicum, seeded and cut into thin strips
2 sticks celery, cut into thin strips
½ cup natural sultanas
¼ cup herb vinegar
1 tablespoon olive oil
1 teaspoon curry powder

METHOD
1. Place vegetables and sultanas into a large salad bowl. Toss lightly.
2. Mix vinegar, oil and curry powder together in a small bowl. Pour dressing over Cauliflower Salad.

Serves 6.

HOT BEAN SALAD

INGREDIENTS

125 g (4 ozs) young green beans
½ cup almond slivers
1 tomato, cut into small dice
½ cup chopped shallots
1 medium carrot, peeled and finely grated
1 small zucchini, cut into small dice
½ cup finely chopped celery
½ teaspoon mustard
125 g (4 ozs) firm tofu, cut into small dice

METHOD

1. Top and tail beans and remove any strings. Cut beans into small pieces.
2. *Convection Cookery.* Place beans into a steamer and cook until just tender.
   or
   Microwave Cookery. Place beans onto a large flat microwave-safe plate. Cover with vented plastic wrap. Microwave on high for approx. 3 minutes or until just tender.
3. Toast almond slivers under a hot griller.
4. Place all the ingredients except mustard and tofu into a medium sized mixing bowl and stir well.
5. *Convection Cookery.* Place ingredients into a non-stick frying pan and cook over a gentle heat, stirring occasionally until heated through.
   or
   Microwave Cookery. Place ingredients into a microwave-safe dish. Microwave on high for approx. 5 minutes or until heated through, stirring occasionally during heating.
6. Stir mustard and tofu into bean salad just before serving.

Serves 4-6 as a side salad.

HOT POTATO SALAD

This potato salad is a delicious accompaniment to fish or meat dishes. It has no added salt or fat.

INGREDIENTS
6 medium-large sized potatoes
juice of 1 lemon
1 tablespoon concentrated apple juice
  (no added sugar)
1 tablespoon white vinegar
1 clove garlic, peeled and crushed
2 tablespoons finely chopped fresh parsley
½ teaspoon dried salad herbs (of your choice)
½ cup finely chopped shallots
¼ cup finely chopped green capsicum
1 stalk celery, finely chopped

METHOD
1. Prepare a large flat convection or microwave-safe casserole dish by spraying with cooking spray.
2. Peel potatoes and cut into dice.
3. *Convection Cookery.* Place potato into a steamer and steam until just tender.
or

   Microwave Cookery. Place potato onto a large flat microwave-safe plate. Cover with vented plastic. Microwave on high for approx. 8 minutes or until potato is just tender.
4. While potato is cooking, prepare dressing by mixing lemon juice, apple juice, vinegar, garlic, parsley and herbs together in a 1 litre (2 pt) jug.
5. Place cooked potato into prepared casserole dish.
6. Mix shallots, capsicum and celery together and sprinkle over cooked potato.
7. Pour dressing over salad.

Serves 6-8.

WALDORF CHICKEN SALAD

This is an excellent salad to serve at a barbecue. It provides an alternative for those who choose to cut down on red meat. Serve in lettuce cups or as desired.

INGREDIENTS
½ cup quick brown rice
1½ cups warm water
1 teaspoon mustard
½ cup mashed tofu
2 cups cooked diced chicken
  (all skin and fat removed)
1½ cups finely sliced celery
1 cup green grapes, cut in half and seeds removed
1 cup black grapes, cut in half and seeds removed
1 large green apple, cored and cut into small dice
1 large red apple, cored and cut into small dice
½ cup chopped walnuts

METHOD
1. *Convection Cookery.* Place rice and water into a medium sized saucepan. Cook with lid off until rice is tender.
or
   Microwave Cookery. Place rice and water into a large microwave-safe bowl. Microwave on high for approx. 8 minutes or until rice is tender.
2. Strain any remaining liquid from rice and place rice into a large serving bowl.
3. Stir mustard into tofu.
4. Add remaining ingredients to serving bowl. Gently stir in mustard-tofu.

Serves 6.

ZUCCHINI SALAD

Healthy and nutritious vegetable salads make a good addition to any meal.

INGREDIENTS
2 cups grated zucchini
½ cup finely chopped red capsicum
½ cup finely chopped green capsicum
1 cup chopped celery
¼ cup finely chopped walnuts
2 tablespoons finely chopped fresh parsley

METHOD
1. Mix all the ingredients together and serve in a suitable salad bowl.

Serves 6.

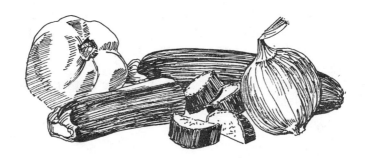

DESSERTS

	MILK-FREE	WHEAT-FREE	EGG-FREE	LOW-FAT	LOW-SUGAR	CONVECTION	MICROWAVE	FREEZER
Apricot Supreme	•	•	•	•		•		•
Apple Crumble	•		•	•		•	•	•
Banana Wraps	•		•	•	•	•		
Mango Ice	•	•	•	•	•			•
Oranges with Snow	•	•		•		•		
Sorbet	•	•		•		•	•	•
Soya-Cottage Peaches	•	•	•	•	•	•	•	
Tofu Ice-cream	•	•			•			•

Desserts

The desserts in this section are all designed to be low in fat. It is very important that we remember Australian Dietary Guideline No. 3 to reduce the fat intake in our diet. There is no point in following a healthy diet if a healthy main meal is followed by a fattening dessert.

APRICOT SUPREME

This dessert is so named because it is a superb finale at a dinner party. The apricots may be served hot or cold as desired.

INGREDIENTS

APRICOTS
500 g (1 lb) dried apricots
6 cups boiling water
1 cup orange juice
2 tablespoons maize cornflour
3 tablespoons cold water

CARAMEL-ORANGE SAUCE
1 cup sugar
⅓ cup warm water
½ cup boiling water
juice and finely grated rind of 1 orange
2 tablespoons Grand Marnier liqueur
1 tablespoon maize cornflour
2 tablespoons cold water

METHOD

APRICOTS
1.   Place apricots into a large bowl.
2.   Pour boiling water and orange juice over apricots.
3.   Seal and leave overnight.
4.   Next day, pour apricots and liquid into a large saucepan and bring to the boil.
5.   Place cornflour into a small bowl. Add a little cold water and blend well. Stir in remaining cold water.
6.   Pour blended cornflour into apricots and return to the boil. Cook for 2 minutes, stirring continuously.
7.   Pour into serving bowls.
8.   Prepare Caramel-Orange Sauce.

CARAMEL-ORANGE SAUCE

1. Place sugar and warm water into a small saucepan.
2. Stir over a low heat until sugar dissolves.
3. Increase heat and boil rapidly until mixture is a pale honey colour. Take care not to burn syrup. Remove from heat.
4. Carefully pour in the boiling water, orange juice, orange rind and Grand Marnier.
5. Place cornflour into a small bowl. Add a little cold water and blend well. Stir in remaining water. Pour into saucepan.
6. Stir over a gentle heat until sauce boils and thickens.
7. Pour sauce over apricots.

Serves 6-8.

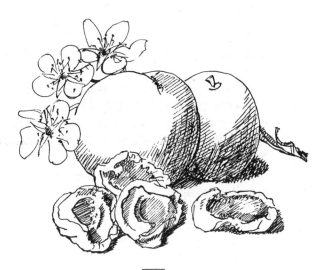

APPLE CRUMBLE

Apple Crumble has been a popular dessert for many years. It is delicious served warm or cold with soy-custard.

INGREDIENTS
6 large green cooking apples
1 piece of lemon peel
6 whole cloves
1 cup Kellogg's* All-Bran†
1 cup wholemeal self-raising flour
1 tablespoon soft polyunsaturated margarine (milk-free)
1 teaspoon cinnamon
¼ cup raw sugar

METHOD
1. Peel and core apples and cut into small dice.
2. *Convection Cookery.* Place apple into a steamer. Add lemon peel and cloves and cook until tender.
   or
   Microwave Cookery. Place apple into a large microwave-safe dish. Add lemon peel and cloves. Cover with vented plastic wrap. Microwave on high for approx. 8 minutes or until apple is tender.
3. Remove lemon peel and cloves.
4. Preheat oven to 200°C (400°F).
5. Prepare a 30 cm x 23 cm (12″ x 9″) dish by spraying with cooking spray.
6. Spread cooked apple over base of prepared dish.
7. Mix remaining ingredients together and spread evenly over apple.
8. Bake for approx. 10-15 minutes or until topping is golden brown as desired.

Serves 6.

BANANA WRAPS

These Banana Wraps are ideal for a low cholesterol, low-fat diet as filo pastry, which is low in fat, is used. You can make up as many or as few wraps as you like, depending on the number of bananas you use.

INGREDIENTS
bananas
filo pastry sheets
finely chopped green ginger
brown sugar

METHOD
1. Preheat oven to 200°C (400°F).
2. Prepare a flat oven tray by spraying with cooking spray.
3. Peel bananas and cut in half lengthwise and crosswise (4 pieces from each banana).
4. Place quarter of a banana onto half a sheet of filo pastry.
5. Add a few pieces of ginger and half a teaspoon of brown sugar.
6. Wrap up well. Wrap again in another half sheet of filo pastry.
7. Bake for approx. 15 minutes or until golden brown.

Serve warm or cold as desired.

MANGO ICE

This is a very refreshing dessert to serve at the end of a meal.

INGREDIENTS
4 ripe mangoes
1 cup soy drink

METHOD
1. Peel and slice mangoes
2. Place mango flesh into the bowl of an electric food processor or blender and blend until smooth.
3. Stir in soy drink.
4. Pour into a flat tray and freeze until just beginning to set.
5. Place into a bowl and whip with an electric mixer.
6. Pour into a flat tray and freeze until required.
7. Thaw a little before serving.

Serves 6.

ORANGES WITH SNOW

Today we tend to look for dessert recipes that are low in fat. This recipe is easy to prepare and will delight the palate of those who enjoy oranges with brandy.

INGREDIENTS

3 large sweet oranges
¼ cup finely chopped natural dried raisins
3 tablespoons brandy
1 tablespoon sugar
3 egg whites
3 tablespoons castor sugar

METHOD

1. Cut oranges in half and scoop out flesh. Reserve orange skins in a sealed container and place into refrigerator.
2. Chop orange flesh and place into an airtight container. Add raisins, brandy and sugar. Seal and marinate in refrigerator overnight (optional).
3. Next day, preheat oven to 230°C (450°F).
4. Fill orange shells with marinated fruit. Take care not to over-fill shells, to allow room for meringue topping.
5. Place orange shells onto a flat oven tray. Steady orange shells with balls of foil if necessary. Place into freezer for 10 minutes.
6. In a separate, clean, dry bowl, beat egg whites until stiff. Gradually add castor sugar, beating well to make a stiff meringue.
7. Remove filled orange shells from freezer and pile meringue on top of each.
8. Bake for only a few minutes until peaks are just lightly brown.
9. Serve warm or cool as desired.

Serves 6.

SORBET

When the occasion arises to have guests who are unaccustomed to a low fat, low salt or low sugar diet, it is difficult for the host or hostess to choose a dessert that will please their palate and at the same time not wander too far away from a healthy diet. Sorbets are desserts that will help you out in this situation. They are easy to prepare and can be prepared ahead of time and stored in the freezer until required.

ORANGE SORBET

INGREDIENTS
1 cup water
2 tablespoons sugar
200 ml (7 fl ozs) concentrated orange juice
  (no added sugar)
1 tablespoon Grand Marnier liqueur
1 egg white

METHOD
1. *Convection Cookery.* Place water and sugar into a small saucepan. Bring to the boil.
    or
    Microwave Cookery. Place water and sugar into a small microwave-safe bowl. Microwave on high for approx. 1 minute or until syrup boils.
2. Allow to cool.
3. Stir in orange juice and Grand Marnier.
4. Pour into a shallow tray and freeze until just beginning to set.
5. Stir with a fork to mix evenly.

6. In a separate, clean, dry bowl, beat egg white until stiff and lightly fold into mixture.
7. Return to tray and freeze until required.

Serves 4.

STRAWBERRY SORBET

If you wish to improve the flavour of this dessert the strawberries can be prepared and soaked with the gin overnight.

INGREDIENTS
1 cup water
⅓ cup sugar
1 punnet strawberries
3 tablespoons gin
½ cup dry white wine
1 egg white

METHOD
1. *Convection Cookery.* Place water and sugar into a small saucepan. Bring to the boil.
or

   Microwave Cookery. Place water and sugar into a small microwave-safe bowl. Microwave on high for approx. 1 minute or until syrup boils.
2. Hull and wash strawberries.
3. Blend syrup, strawberries, gin and wine in the bowl of an electric food processor or blender or rub through a sieve or Mouli.
4. Pour into a shallow tray and freeze until just beginning to set.
5. Stir with a fork to mix evenly.
6. In a separate, clean, dry bowl, beat egg white until stiff and lightly fold into mixture.
7. Return to tray and freeze until required.

Serves 6.

LEMON SORBET

INGREDIENTS
½ cup water
¼ cup sugar
½ cup white wine
½ cup lemon juice
1 egg white

METHOD
1. *Convection Cookery.* Place water and sugar into a small saucepan. Bring to the boil.

   or

   Microwave Cookery. Place water and sugar into a small microwave-safe bowl. Microwave on high for approx. 1 minute or until syrup boils.
2. Allow to cool.
3. Stir in wine and lemon juice.
4. Pour into a shallow tray and freeze until just beginning to set.
5. Stir with a fork to mix evenly.
6. In a separate, clean, dry bowl, beat egg white until stiff and lightly fold into mixture.
7. Return to tray and freeze until required.

Serves 4.

APPLE SORBET

This sorbet contains no added sugar. It is very easy to prepare as no cooking is required.

INGREDIENTS
1 cup concentrated apple juice (no added sugar)
¼ cup white wine
1 egg white

METHOD
1. Pour apple juice and wine into a shallow tray and freeze until just beginning to set.
2. Stir with a fork to mix evenly.
3. In a separate, clean, dry bowl, beat egg white until stiff and lightly fold into mixture.
4. Return to tray and freeze until required.

Serves 2-3.

GRAPE SORBET

This sorbet contains no added sugar. It is very easy to prepare as no cooking is required. Two tablespoons of port can be added, if desired.

INGREDIENTS
1 cup grape juice (no added sugar)
2 tablespoons port (optional)
1 egg white

METHOD
1. Pour grape juice and port (if desired), into a shallow tray and freeze until just beginning to set.
2. Stir with a fork to mix evenly.
3. In a separate, clean, dry bowl, beat egg white until stiff and lightly fold into mixture.
4. Return to tray and freeze until required.

Serves 2-3.

SOYA-COTTAGE PEACHES

This is a very delicious low-fat dessert. It can be prepared in the morning and served in the evening. The number of peaches can be increased for a larger number of guests. If fresh peaches are not available canned peach halves in natural juice can be used. If using canned peaches, omit steps 2 and 3 and pour ¼ cup natural juice over peaches.

INGREDIENTS
½ cup almond flakes
6 large ripe peaches, peeled and cut in half
¼ cup water
1 tablespoon brown sugar
250 g (8 ozs) soya cottage cheese
a few drops almond essence
¼ teaspoon vanilla essence
½ cup icing sugar mixture
1 tablespoon raw sugar
½ cup boiling water
1 cup orange juice
⅓ cup brandy
½ cup Grand Marnier liqueur
2 tablespoons maize cornflour
2 tablespoons cold water

METHOD
1. Place almond flakes onto a flat oven tray. Toast under a hot griller until golden brown. Take care not to burn almond flakes.
2. *Convection Cookery.* Place peaches into a large flat pan with a lid. Pour water over peaches. Sprinkle peaches with brown sugar. Bring to the boil and boil for 1 minute with the lid on. Remove from heat.
    or

Microwave Cookery. Place peaches over the base of a large flat microwave-safe dish. Pour water over peaches. Sprinkle peaches with brown sugar. Cover with vented plastic wrap and microwave on high for 3 minutes.

3. Allow peaches to cool and refrigerate until cold.
4. Place soya cottage cheese into a small mixing bowl. Add almond essence, vanilla essence and icing sugar and mix well.
5. Place approx. 1 tablespoon soya cottage cheese mixture into each peach half. Return to the refrigerator.
6. Place sugar and boiling water into a small saucepan.
7. Stir over a low heat until sugar dissolves.
8. Increase heat and boil rapidly until syrup is a pale honey colour. Take care not to burn the syrup.
9. Remove from heat and carefully pour in orange juice, brandy and Grand Marnier.
10. Place cornflour into a small bowl. Add a little cold water and blend well. Stir in remaining water. Pour into saucepan.
11. Stir over a gentle heat until sauce boils and thickens. Set sauce aside until required for serving.
12. To serve — arrange one or two filled peach halves in individual serving dishes. Serve with sauce and toasted almond flakes.

Serves 6 or 12 depending on size of peaches.

TOFU ICE-CREAM

Milk-free ice-cream can be delicious. This recipe is made with tofu. Flavours such as carob, mashed banana, caramel or honey can be added as desired. This ice-cream freezes very hard and is best taken out of the freezer half an hour before it is required, or it can be softened in the microwave.

INGREDIENTS
375 g (12 ozs) cold soft tofu
1 litre (32 fl ozs) cold soy drink
1 tablespoon gelatine
2 tablespoons water   ·
1 teaspoon vanilla essence
2 egg whites
½ cup castor sugar

METHOD
1. Rub tofu through a fine sieve.
2. Blend tofu and 500 ml (16 fl ozs) soy drink in an electric food processor or blender.
3. Dissolve gelatine in water. Heat over a low heat until boiling. Stir into tofu-soy mixture.
4. Freeze until just beginning to set.
5. Whip icy mixture with the remaining 500 ml (16 fl ozs) cold soy drink and vanilla.
6. In a separate, clean, dry bowl, beat egg whites until stiff. Gradually add sugar and beat to a stiff meringue. Fold into ice-cream mixture.
7. Freeze until required.

Makes approx. 4 litres (6 pints).

HEALTHY GOODIES TO BAKE

	MILK-FREE	WHEAT-FREE	EGG-FREE	LOW-FAT	LOW-SUGAR	CONVECTION	MICROWAVE	FREEZER
BISCUITS								
Honey Biscuits	•					•		•
Honey-Bran Biscuits	•		•			•		•
Pecan Biscuits	•					•		•
Walnut Biscuits	•					•		•
BREAD								
Bran Bread	•			•		•	•	•
Corn Bread	•		•		•	•		•
Great Australian Damper	•		•	•		•	•	•
Wholemeal Bread	•		•	•	•	•	•	•
Wholemeal Buns	•		•			•		•
CAKES AND SLICES								
Apple-Fruit Cake	•		•			•		•
Banana Cake	•		•			•		•
Carrot-Pineapple Cake	•		•			•		•
Marmalade Bars	•		•			•		•
Orange Slice	•					•		•
Pineapple Cake	•					•		•
Pumpkin-Sultana Cake	•					•		•

	MILK-FREE	WHEAT-FREE	EGG-FREE	LOW-FAT	LOW-SUGAR	CONVECTION	MICROWAVE	FREEZER
LOAVES								
Apricot Bran Loaf	•			•		•		•
Date and Ginger Loaf	•		•	•		•		•
Fruit Loaf	•			•		•	•	•
Irish Bambrack	•			•		•		•
Sultana-Grape Loaf	•		•	•		•		•
MUFFINS								
Apple and Oat Bran Muffins	•		•			•		•
Boysenberry Muffins	•	•				•		•
Fruit Muffins	•		•	•		•		•
Oat Bran and Ginger Muffins	•					•		•

Healthy Goodies to Bake

It is very important that the cakes and slices we eat are healthy. There is no reason why we have to remove these items from our diet. It is important to reduce fat and sugar levels and include wholemeal products wherever possible.

All the recipes in this section use wholemeal flour. If you wish to, you can substitute white flour, however it is important to note the nutritional and fibre benefits of wholemeal flour.

It is also important to use common sense on a low-fat diet and to limit intake to 1 piece of cake or muffin, or 2 small biscuits per serving. Low-fat recipes such as Bran Bread on page 138-9 can be consumed in place of cake if a very strict low-fat diet is required.

HONEY BISCUITS

INGREDIENTS

125 g (4 ozs) polyunsaturated margarine
(milk-free)
125 g (4 ozs) raw sugar
2 tablespoons honey
1 egg
½ teaspoon vanilla essence
1 cup Sunfarm rice bran
1 teaspoon baking powder
2 cups wholemeal self-raising flour
½ cup sunflower seed kernels

METHOD

1. Preheat oven to 160°C (325°F).
2. Prepare 2 flat heatproof oven trays by spraying with cooking spray.
3. Cream margarine, sugar, honey, egg and vanilla.
4. Stir bran into creamed mixture.
5. Stir baking powder into flour. Add to creamed mixture and mix well.
6. Place sunflower seed kernels onto a flat heatproof tray. Toast under a hot griller. Stir into creamed mixture.
7. Using lightly floured hands, roll into balls approx. the size of a walnut.
8. Place onto prepared trays.
9. Carefully flatten with a fork dipped in flour.
10. Bake for approx. 15 minutes or until golden brown and cooked.
11. When cooked, remove from oven and leave on trays for 2 minutes. Loosen biscuits and leave on trays to cool.
12. When completely cold, store in an airtight container.

Makes approx. 40 biscuits.

HONEY-BRAN BISCUITS

Fibre is a very important part of our diet. With this in mind, two different types of bran and wholemeal flour are used in this recipe.

INGREDIENTS
1 cup Sunfarm rice bran
1 cup Kellogg's* All-Bran†
1 cup wholemeal self-raising flour
⅓ cup sugar
*125 g (4 ozs) polyunsaturated margarine
  (milk-free)*
1 tablespoon honey
½ teaspoon vanilla essence

METHOD
1. Preheat oven to 160°C (325°F).
2. Prepare a flat oven tray by spraying with cooking spray.
3. Place rice bran, All-Bran, flour and sugar into a medium sized mixing bowl.
4. Melt margarine. Stir in honey and vanilla. Warm gently to soften honey.
5. Make a well in the centre of the dry ingredients. Pour in liquid and mix well.
6. Place heaped teaspoons of mixture onto prepared tray.
7. Bake for approx. 15 minutes or until golden brown and cooked.
8. When cooked, remove from oven and leave on tray for 2 minutes. Loosen biscuits and leave on tray to cool.
9. When completely cold, store in an airtight container.

Makes approx. 18 biscuits.

PECAN BISCUITS

Walnuts can be substituted for pecans in this recipe if desired.

INGREDIENTS
90 g (3 ozs) polyunsaturated margarine (milk-free)
¼ cup raw sugar
2 tablespoons honey
1 egg
½ teaspoon vanilla essence
½ cup Kellogg's* All-Bran†
½ teaspoon baking powder
1 teaspoon mixed spice
1¼ cups wholemeal flour
½ cup finely chopped pecans

METHOD
1. Preheat oven to 160°C (325°F).
2. Prepare a large flat oven tray by spraying with cooking spray.
3. Cream margarine, sugar, honey, egg and vanilla.
4. Stir All-Bran into creamed mixture.
5. Stir baking powder and spice into wholemeal flour. Add to creamed mixture and mix well.
6. Stir in pecans.
7. Place heaped teaspoons of mixture onto prepared tray. Carefully flatten with a fork dipped in flour.
8. Bake for approx. 15 minutes or until golden brown and cooked.
9. When cooked, remove from oven and leave on tray for 2 minutes. Loosen biscuits and leave on tray to cool.
10. When completely cold, store in an airtight container.

Makes approx. 24 biscuits.

WALNUT BISCUITS

These biscuits are high in fibre and low in fat and sugar. They are good for lunch-box cookies. Other crunchy bran products such as Sunfarm rice bran can be substituted for All-Bran.

INGREDIENTS
2 tablespoons polyunsaturated margarine (milk-free)
2 tablespoons raw sugar
1 egg
1 teaspoon vanilla essence
½ cup Kellogg's* All-Bran†
½ cup natural dried sultanas
¼ cup finely chopped walnuts
½ cup wholemeal flour
½ cup wholemeal self-raising flour

METHOD
1. Preheat oven to 160°C (325°F).
2. Prepare a large flat oven tray by spraying with cooking spray.
3. Cream margarine, sugar, egg and vanilla.
4. Stir All-Bran, sultanas, walnuts and flours into creamed mixture.
5. Mix to a firm dough.
6. Using lightly floured hands, roll into balls approx. the size of a walnut.
7. Place onto prepared tray. Carefully flatten with a fork dipped in flour.
8. Bake for approx. 15 minutes or until golden brown and cooked.
9. When cooked, remove from oven and leave on

tray for 2 minutes. Loosen biscuits and leave on tray to cool.
10. When completely cold, store in an airtight container.

Makes approx. 24 biscuits.

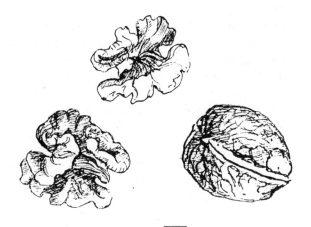

BRAN BREAD

This is a high-fibre, fruit and bran bread. It is delicious served warm.

INGREDIENTS
1 tablespoon polyunsaturated margarine (milk-free)
1½ cups warm water
2 tablespoons honey
2 x 7 g sachets dried yeast
1 egg, lightly beaten
3 cups wholemeal flour
1 cup Kellogg's* All-Bran†
1 teaspoon cinnamon
1 cup chopped natural dried sultanas

METHOD
1. Prepare a flat oven tray by spraying with cooking spray.
2. Melt margarine and pour into a large mixing bowl.
3. Add water, honey and yeast and stir well.
4. Allow to stand in a warm place for approx. 10 minutes or until frothy.
5. Stir in egg.
6. Place flour into a large ovenproof or microwave-safe bowl.
7. *Convection Cookery*. Preheat oven to 100°C (200°F). Warm flour for 5 minutes.
or

   Microwave Cookery. Microwave flour on high for 1 minute.
8. Add warmed flour, All-Bran, cinnamon and sultanas to liquid and mix well.
9. Cover and place in a warm position to prove until double in size (approx. 20 minutes).

10. Turn dough out onto a lightly floured board and knead well.
11. Shape as desired.
12. Place onto prepared tray.
13. Place in a warm position for approx. 20 minutes or until bread springs back when touched.
14. Preheat oven to 200°C (400°F).
15. Bake for approx. 20 minutes or until golden brown and cooked when tested.

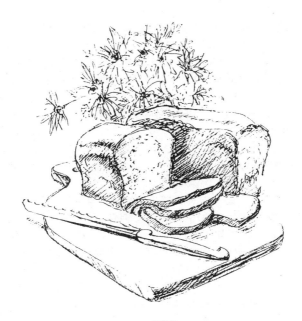

CORN BREAD

High fibre breads are a valuable addition to any diet.

INGREDIENTS
1½ cups wholemeal self-raising flour
3 teaspoons baking powder
½ teaspoon cayenne pepper
100 g (3½ ozs) polyunsaturated margarine
   (milk-free)
¾ cup polenta
1 tablespoon castor sugar
2 tablespoons finely chopped fresh parsley
1 onion, peeled and finely chopped
1¼ cups water

METHOD
1.   Preheat oven to 220°C (425°F).
2.   Prepare a flat oven tray by spraying with cooking spray.
3.   Place flour, baking powder and cayenne pepper into a medium sized mixing bowl. Rub margarine into dry ingredients until mixture resembles fine breadcrumbs. This process may be done by hand or with the aid of an electric food processor.
4.   Stir polenta, sugar, parsley and onion into dry ingredients.
5.   Make a well in the centre of the dry ingredients and pour in water.
6.   Mix to a firm dough.
7.   Using lightly floured hands, shape into a loaf and place onto prepared tray.
8.   Bake for approx. 20 minutes or until golden brown and cooked when tested.
9.   When cooked, remove from oven and leave on tray for 10 minutes before placing loaf onto a fine wire rack to cool.

GREAT AUSTRALIAN DAMPER

INGREDIENTS

4 cups wholemeal self-raising flour
1 tablespoon sesame or poppy seeds or sunflower
  seed kernels
1 cup chopped natural dried sultanas
1 tablespoon canola oil
1 tablespoon golden syrup
2 cups soy drink
¼ cup wheat germ

METHOD

1. Preheat oven to 220°C (425°F).
2. Prepare a flat oven tray with cooking spray.
3. Place flour into a large bowl.
4. Add seeds and sultanas.
5. *Convection Cookery.* Place oil, golden syrup and soy drink into a small saucepan and heat until just warm.
   Microwave Cookery. Place oil, golden syrup and soy drink into a small microwave-safe bowl. Microwave on high for approx. 40 seconds or until just warm.
6. Make a well in the centre of the dry ingredients and pour in liquid.
7. Mix to a firm dough.
8. Spread wheat germ onto a board.
9. Turn dough out onto wheat germ and knead lightly.
10. Shape into a damper.
11. Place onto prepared tray.
12. Bake for 12 minutes. Reduce heat to 200°C (400°F) and continue to bake for a further 25 minutes approx. or until cooked when tested.
13. When cooked, remove from oven and leave on tray for 5 minutes before placing onto a fine wire rack to cool.

WHOLEMEAL BREAD

This bread is high in fibre as it is made with wholemeal flour.

INGREDIENTS
2 tablespoons canola oil
500 ml (16 fl ozs) warm water
2 x 7 g sachets dried yeast
1 tablespoon raw sugar
1 kg (2 lb) wholemeal flour

METHOD
1. Prepare a large flat oven tray or tins by spraying with cooking spray.
2. Pour oil into a large mixing bowl. Stir in water.
3. Add yeast and sugar to bowl and stir well.
4. Allow to stand in a warm place for approx. 10 minutes or until frothy.
5. Place flour into a large ovenproof or microwave-safe bowl.
6. *Convection Cookery.* Preheat oven to 100°C (200°F). Warm flour for 5 minutes.

    or

    Microwave Cookery. Microwave flour on high for 1 minute.
7. Add warmed flour to liquid and mix well.
8. Cover and place in a warm position to prove until double in size (approx. 20 minutes).
9. Turn dough out onto a lightly floured board and knead well.
10. Shape as desired.
11. Place onto prepared tray or into prepared tins.
12. Place in a warm position for approx. 20 minutes or until bread springs back when touched.
13. Preheat oven to 220°C (425°F).

142

14. *Small loaves:* Bake for approx. 12 minutes or until golden brown and cooked when tested.
    Large loaf: Bake for 12 minutes, reduce heat to 200°C (400°F) and bake for a further 20 minutes approx. or until golden brown and cooked when tested.
15. When cooked, remove from oven and leave on tray or in tins for 5 minutes before turning out onto a fine wire rack to cool.

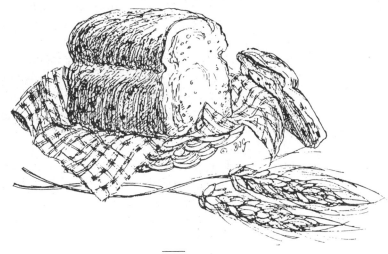

WHOLEMEAL BUNS

These buns are cooked in a very interesting shape. Small terra-cotta garden pots are used for the cooking process. New pots must be soaked in warm water overnight before they can be used.

INGREDIENTS
SCONE DOUGH
2 tablespoons polyunsaturated margarine
   (milk-free)
2 cups wholemeal self-raising flour
1 cup water

SULTANA FILLING
1 tablespoon polyunsaturated margarine (milk-free)
1 tablespoon brown sugar
½ teaspoon vanilla essence
1 cup chopped natural dried sultanas

METHOD
SCONE DOUGH
1. Preheat oven to 200°C (400°F).
2. Prepare 4 x 8 cm (3″) terra-cotta pots by spraying with cooking spray.
3. Rub margarine into flour until mixture resembles fine breadcrumbs. This process may be done by hand or with the aid of an electric food processor.
4. Make a well in the centre of the dry ingredients and pour in water.
5. Mix to a firm dough.
6. Turn dough out onto a lightly floured board and knead lightly.
7. Divide into 4 portions. Roll each portion into a 20 cm (8″) square (approx.).
8. Prepare Sultana Filling.

SULTANA FILLING

1. Place margarine, sugar and vanilla into a small bowl and mix well. Add sultanas and mix well.
2. Place one quarter of Sultana Filling into the centre of each square.
3. Fold up into a small parcel shape. Take care not to stretch the dough during folding.
4. Shape parcels to be slightly narrower at one end and ease one parcel into each pot.
5. Place pots onto a flat oven tray to facilitate handling.
6. Place into oven and bake for approx. 25 minutes or until golden brown and cooked when tested.
7. When cooked, remove from oven and leave in pots for 5 minutes before turning out onto a fine wire rack to cool.

Makes 4 buns.

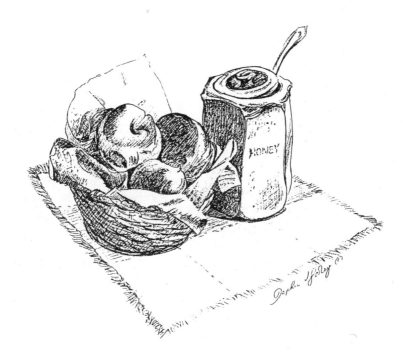

APPLE-FRUIT CAKE

This cake is full of nature's goodness.

INGREDIENTS
60 g (2 ozs) polyunsaturated margarine (milk-free)
60 g (2 ozs) raw sugar
1 teaspoon vanilla essence
2 teaspoons bicarbonate of soda
*1½ cups cold unsweetened cooked apple, drained
(approx. 2 large green cooking apples)*
½ cup finely chopped walnuts
1 cup natural dried raisins (cut in half)
1 cup chopped dates
1 teaspoon cinnamon
1 teaspoon cocoa
½ teaspoon nutmeg
1½ cups wholemeal self-raising flour

METHOD
1. Preheat oven to 180°C (350°F).
2. Prepare a 23 cm x 13 cm (9" x 5") loaf tin by spraying with cooking spray.
3. Cream margarine, sugar and vanilla.
4. Stir bicarbonate of soda into cooked apple. Stir into creamed mixture.
5. Stir in walnuts, raisins and dates.
6. Stir cinnamon, cocoa and nutmeg into flour. Stir into creamed apple mixture.
7. Spread into prepared tin.
8. Bake for approx. 40 minutes or until golden brown and cooked when tested.
9. When cooked, remove from oven and leave in tin for 15 minutes before turning out onto a fine wire rack to cool.

BANANA CAKE

Banana cake is one of my favourite cakes. This is a healthy version of the traditional cake recipe. It is important to use very ripe bananas for the best results.

INGREDIENTS
90 g (3 ozs) polyunsaturated margarine (milk-free)
90 g (3 ozs) brown sugar
1 tablespoon treacle
1 teaspoon vanilla essence
3 ripe bananas
1 Weet-Bix, crushed
1½ cups wholemeal self-raising flour
½ cup soy drink

METHOD
1. Preheat oven to 180°C (350°F).
2. Prepare a 20 cm (8″) fluted ring cake tin by spraying with cooking spray.
3. Cream margarine, sugar, treacle and vanilla.
4. Mash bananas well and stir into creamed mixture.
5. Stir in Weet-Bix.
6. Add flour and soy drink alternately to creamed mixture, stirring well after each addition.
7. Spread into prepared tin.
8. Bake for approx. 45 minutes or until cooked when tested.
9. When cooked, remove from oven and leave in tin for 15 minutes before turning out onto a fine wire rack to cool.

CARROT-PINEAPPLE CAKE

This delicious cake is very moist. It will be enjoyed by those who like a ginger flavour. If you do not like ginger, the cake can be made without it. The cake requires very little mixing; only a few strokes are needed to combine the ingredients.

INGREDIENTS
1½ cups wholemeal self-raising flour
1 teaspoon bicarbonate of soda
½ cup raw sugar
1 teaspoon cinnamon
1 teaspoon ground ginger
⅓ cup canola oil
1 cup grated carrot
1 x 440 g can crushed pineapple (in natural juice)
1 teaspoon vanilla essence
½ cup finely chopped pecans
1 tablespoon chopped green ginger

METHOD
1. Preheat oven to 180°C (350°F).
2. Prepare a 20 cm (8") round cake tin by spraying with cooking spray. Line base of tin with greaseproof paper and spray again.
3. Place all the ingredients into a large bowl.
4. Stir just enough to combine ingredients.
5. Pour into prepared tin.
6. Bake for approx. 45 minutes or until cooked when tested.
7. When cooked, remove from oven and leave in tin for 15 minutes before turning out onto a fine wire rack to cool.

MARMALADE BARS

A crunchy slice with a marmalade and rolled oats topping.

INGREDIENTS
60 g (2 ozs) polyunsaturated margarine (milk-free)
60 g (2ozs) brown sugar
1 teaspoon vanilla essence
1 tablespoon soy drink
1 teaspoon baking powder
1 cup Kellogg's* All-Bran†
¾ cup wholemeal flour
2 tablespoons marmalade
¾ cup rolled oats

METHOD
1. Preheat oven to 180°C (350°F).
2. Prepare a 28 cm x 20 cm (11″ x 8″) slice tin by spraying with cooking spray.
3. Cream margarine, sugar, vanilla and soy drink.
4. Stir baking powder and All-Bran into flour. Mix into creamed mixture.
5. Press into prepared tin.
6. Mix marmalade and rolled oats and spread evenly over mixture in tin.
7. Bake for approx. 20 minutes or until golden brown.
8. While still warm cut into squares and leave in tin to cool.

ORANGE SLICE

This slice has a lovely orange flavour. It is topped with an orange flavoured meringue. It is best kept in the refrigerator if you wish to keep it for more than a couple of days.

INGREDIENTS
ORANGE SLICE
60 g (2 ozs) polyunsaturated margarine (milk-free)
2 cups wholemeal self-raising flour
finely grated rind of ½ orange
½ cup brown sugar
1 egg
1 teaspoon vanilla essence
⅓ cup orange juice
ORANGE MERINGUE TOPPING
30 g (1 oz) almond flakes
2 egg whites
2 tablespoons castor sugar
1 teaspoon vanilla essence
finely grated rind of ½ orange

METHOD
ORANGE SLICE
1. Preheat oven to 180°C (350°F).
2. Prepare a 28 cm x 20 cm (11" x 8") slice tray by spraying with cooking spray.
3. Rub margarine into flour until mixture resembles fine breadcrumbs. This process may be done by hand or with the aid of an electric food processor.
4. Stir in orange rind and sugar.
5. Beat egg and stir in vanilla and orange juice. Mix into dry ingredients.
6. Press mixture into prepared tray.
7. Prepare Orange Meringue Topping.

ORANGE MERINGUE TOPPING

1. Place almond flakes onto a flat oven tray. Toast under a hot griller until golden brown. Take care not to burn almond flakes.
2. In a separate, clean, dry bowl, beat egg whites until stiff. Lightly fold in almond flakes and remaining ingredients.
3. Spread over Orange Slice in tray.
4. Bake for approx. 30 minutes or until firm and golden brown.
5. When cooked, remove from oven and allow to cool slightly. While still warm, cut into squares. Allow to cool in tray.

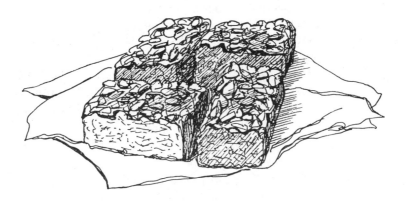

PINEAPPLE CAKE

This is a very moist cake that is best covered and stored in the refrigerator. It can serve eight as a dessert.

INGREDIENTS
PINEAPPLE CAKE
60 g (2 ozs) polyunsaturated margarine (milk-free)
100 g (3½ ozs) raw sugar
1 teaspoon vanilla essence
1 x 440 g can crushed pineapple (in natural juice)
  (reserve 2 tablespoons drained crushed
  pineapple for Pineapple Topping)
2 cups wholemeal self-raising flour
1 egg white

PINEAPPLE TOPPING
250 g (8 ozs) soft tofu
2 tablespoons reserved drained crushed pineapple

METHOD
PINEAPPLE CAKE
1. Preheat oven to 180°C (350°F).
2. Prepare a 20 cm (8″) round cake tin by spraying with cooking spray. Line base of tin with greaseproof paper and spray again.
3. Cream margarine, sugar and vanilla.
4. Stir in pineapple.
5. Stir in flour.
6. In a separate, clean, dry bowl, beat egg white until stiff and lightly fold into mixture.
7. Spread into prepared tin.
8. Bake for approx. 40 minutes or until cooked when tested.
9. When cooked, remove from oven and leave in tin for 15 minutes before turning out onto a fine wire rack to cool.

10. When cold top with Pineapple Topping.

PINEAPPLE TOPPING
1. Rub tofu through a fine sieve.
2. Stir in crushed pineapple.
3. Spread on top of cake.

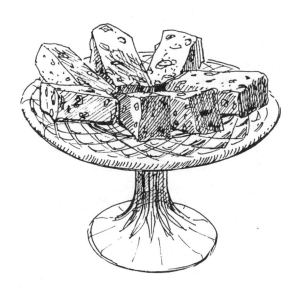

PUMPKIN-SULTANA CAKE

The addition of mashed pumpkin makes a very moist cake. The cake is best stored in the refrigerator, if you wish to keep it for more than a couple of days.

INGREDIENTS

125 g (4 ozs) polyunsaturated margarine (milk-free)
125 g (4 ozs) raw sugar
finely grated rind of 1 orange
1 cup cold cooked mashed pumpkin
1 teaspoon vanilla essence
2 cups chopped natural dried sultanas
½ cup finely chopped walnuts
2 cups wholemeal self-raising flour
2 egg whites

METHOD

1. Preheat oven to 150°C (300°F).
2. Prepare a 23 cm (8″) round cake tin by spraying with cooking spray. Line base of tin with greaseproof paper and spray again.
3. Cream margarine and sugar.
4. Stir in orange rind and pumpkin and beat well.
5. Stir in vanilla, sultanas and walnuts.
6. Add wholemeal flour and mix well.
7. In a separate, clean, dry bowl, beat egg whites until stiff and lightly fold into mixture.
8. Spread into prepared tin.
9. Bake for approx. 50 minutes or until cooked when tested.
10. When cooked, remove from oven and leave in tin for 10 minutes before turning out onto a fine wire rack to cool.

APRICOT BRAN LOAF

This is a very delicious loaf that is sweetened with honey and orange juice. It is excellent in the diet as it is high in fibre.

INGREDIENTS
1 cup Sunfarm rice bran
⅔ cup chopped natural dried sultanas
125 g (4 ozs) dried apricots, finely chopped
¼ cup honey
1½ cups orange juice
1½ cups wholemeal self-raising flour
1 tablespoon canola oil
½ teaspoon bicarbonate of soda
1 egg
½ teaspoon vanilla essence

METHOD
1. Place bran, sultanas, apricots, honey and orange juice into a large bowl and stir well. Cover bowl and allow to stand for at least 2 hours.
2. Preheat oven to 180°C (350°F).
3. Prepare a 23 cm x 9 cm (9" x 3½") loaf tin by spraying with cooking spray.
4. Stir flour into ingredients in bowl.
5. Pour oil into a small bowl. Stir in bicarbonate of soda. Stir into loaf mixture.
6. In a separate, clean, dry bowl, beat egg well. Add vanilla and stir into mixture.
7. Spread mixture into prepared tin.
8. Bake for approx. 45 minutes or until cooked when tested.
9. When cooked, remove from oven and leave in tin for 10 minutes, before turning out onto a fine wire rack to cool.

DATE AND GINGER LOAF

This loaf is very easy to make. It will be sure to please those who like the combination of date and ginger.

INGREDIENTS
1 cup chopped dates
¼ cup concentrated apple juice (no added sugar)
¾ cup boiling water
2 tablespoons brown sugar
1 tablespoon finely chopped green ginger
1½ cups wholemeal self-raising flour
1 teaspoon bicarbonate of soda
1 tablespoon canola oil
½ teaspoon vanilla essence

METHOD
1. Prepare a 23 cm x 9 cm (9" x 3½") loaf tin by spraying with cooking spray.
2. Place chopped dates into a large bowl.
3. Pour in apple juice and boiling water. Allow to stand for 15 minutes.
4. Preheat oven to 180°C (350°F).
5. Add remaining ingredients and stir well.
6. Spread mixture evenly into prepared tin.
7. Bake for approx. 35 minutes or until cooked when tested.
8. When cooked, remove from oven and leave in tin for 15 minutes, before turning out onto a fine wire rack to cool.

IRISH BAMBRACK

This traditional Irish recipe can be made with no added fat. This version has an almond flavour attributable largely to the use of almond tea.

INGREDIENTS

1 cup hot almond tea
1 cup natural dried currants
1 cup chopped natural dried sultanas
½ cup almond slivers
½ cup raw sugar
a few drops of almond essence (as desired)
2 cups wholemeal self-raising flour
1 egg white

METHOD

1. Make tea and allow to infuse for 10 minutes.
2. Place currants, sultanas, almond slivers and sugar into a large bowl. Pour in tea and almond essence and mix well. Seal and leave overnight.
3. Next day — preheat oven to 180°C (350°F).
4. Prepare a 20 cm x 10 cm (8″ x 4″) loaf tin by spraying with cooking spray.
5. Stir flour into soaked fruits and nuts.
6. In a separate, clean, dry bowl, beat egg white until stiff and lightly fold into mixture.
7. Spread into prepared tin.
8. Bake for approx. 50 minutes or until cooked when tested.
9. When cooked, remove from oven and leave in tin for 15 minutes before turning out onto a fine wire rack to cool.

FRUIT LOAF

This is a very nutritious loaf with very little added fat. Honey is added for sweetening instead of sugar.

INGREDIENTS
1 cup Kellogg's* All-Bran†
1 cup chopped natural dried sultanas
1 tablespoon canola oil
¼ cup honey
¾ cup boiling water
1 teaspoon vanilla essence
1 cup wholemeal self-raising flour
1 teaspoon cinnamon
1 teaspoon mixed spice
¼ cup finely chopped walnuts
1 cup grated apple
1 egg white

METHOD
1. Preheat oven to 180°C (350°F) for convection cookery.
2. Prepare a 23 cm x 9 cm (9″ x 3½″) loaf tin for convection cookery or a 23 cm (9″) microwave-safe ring mould by spraying with cooking spray.
3. Mix all the ingredients except the egg white together until well combined.
4. In a separate, clean, dry bowl, beat egg white until stiff and lightly fold into mixture.
5. Spread mixture evenly into prepared tin or mould.
6. *Convection Cookery.* Bake for approx. 40 minutes or until cooked when tested.
or

Microwave Cookery. Microwave on high for

approx. 8 minutes or until cooked when tested.
7. When cooked, remove from oven and leave in tin or mould for 15 minutes before turning out onto a fine wire rack to cool.

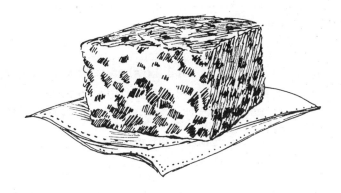

SULTANA-GRAPE LOAF

This loaf uses unsweetened grape juice as the liquid, which gives it a lovely flavour when combined with sultanas.

INGREDIENTS
1 cup Sunfarm rice bran
1 cup chopped natural dried sultanas
2 tablespoons raw sugar
2 tablespoons cream sherry
grape juice (no added sugar)
2 tablespoons honey
1½ cups wholemeal self-raising flour
1 tablespoon polyunsaturated oil
½ teaspoon bicarbonate of soda

METHOD
1. Place bran, sultanas and raw sugar into a bowl.
2. Pour sherry into a 2 cup measure. Add grape juice to make 1⅓ cups liquid.
3. Stir honey into liquid.
4. Pour liquid into dry ingredients in bowl and mix well.
5. Cover bowl and allow to stand for 2 hours.
6. Preheat oven to 180°C (350°F).
7. Prepare a 23 cm x 9 cm (9″ x 3½″) loaf tin by spraying with cooking spray.
8. Stir flour into ingredients in bowl.
9. Pour oil into a small bowl and stir in bicarbonate of soda. Stir into ingredients in bowl and mix well.
10. Spread mixture into prepared tin.
11. Bake for approx. 40 minutes or until cooked when tested.
12. When cooked, remove from oven and leave in tin for 10 minutes before turning out onto a fine wire rack to cool.

160

APPLE AND OAT BRAN MUFFINS

These muffins are light and delicious and are high in fibre.

INGREDIENTS
*125 g (4 ozs) polyunsaturated margarine
    (milk-free)*
²/₃ cup golden syrup
½ teaspoon vanilla essence
1¼ cups wholemeal self-raising flour
½ teaspoon cinnamon
2 teaspoons baking powder
1¼ cups oat bran
½ cup soy drink
1 apple, peeled, cored and finely grated

METHOD
1. Preheat oven to 250°C (475°F).
2. Prepare a muffin tray by spraying with cooking spray.
3. Cream margarine, golden syrup and vanilla.
4. Add remaining ingredients and mix well.
5. Place tablespoons of mixture into prepared muffin tray.
6. Bake for approx. 12 minutes or until golden brown and cooked when tested.
7. When cooked, remove from oven and leave in tray for 5 minutes before placing muffins onto a fine wire rack to cool.

Makes approx. 12 muffins.

BOYSENBERRY MUFFINS

These muffins have a delicious boysenberry flavour. My daughter made up the recipe for afternoon tea one day. The muffins are wheat-free for those who wish to exclude wheat from their diet. Muffin tray paper liners are now available.

INGREDIENTS
180 g (6 ozs) polyunsaturated margarine
 (milk-free)
1 cup castor sugar
½ teaspoon vanilla essence
1 egg, lightly beaten
1½ cups white rice flour
½ cup brown rice flour
½ cup maize cornflour
3 teaspoons baking powder
½ cup Sunfarm rice bran
½ cup polenta
1 cup soy drink
1 x 450 g can boysenberries

METHOD
1. Preheat oven to 250°C (475°F).
2. Prepare 2 muffin trays by spraying with cooking spray.
3. Cream margarine, sugar and vanilla.
4. Add egg and beat well.
5. Sift rice flours, cornflour and baking powder into a medium sized mixing bowl. Stir in rice bran and polenta.
6. Add dry ingredients and soy drink alternately to creamed mixture, mixing well after each addition.
7. Stir in boysenberries.

8. Place tablespoons of mixture into prepared muffin trays.
9. Bake for approx. 12 minutes or until golden brown and cooked when tested.
10. When cooked, remove from oven and leave in tray for 5 minutes before placing muffins onto a fine wire rack to cool.

Makes approx. 22 muffins.

FRUIT MUFFINS

These muffins are high in fibre with a lovely fruity flavour.

INGREDIENTS
1 cup wholemeal self-raising flour
½ cup oat bran
1 teaspoon baking powder
½ cup brown sugar
½ cup chopped dates
1 teaspoon finely grated orange rind
1 banana, well mashed
1 tablespoon finely chopped green ginger
1 tablespoon canola oil
1 cup soy drink
½ teaspoon vanilla essence

METHOD
1. Preheat oven to 250°C (475°F).
2. Prepare a muffin tray by spraying with cooking spray.
3. Place all the ingredients into a large bowl and mix well.
4. Place tablespoons of mixture into prepared muffin tray.
5. Bake for approx. 12 minutes or until golden brown and cooked when tested.
6. When cooked, remove from oven and leave in tray for 5 minutes before placing muffins onto a fine wire rack to cool.

Makes approx. 12 muffins.

OAT BRAN AND GINGER MUFFINS

INGREDIENTS

*125 g (4 ozs) polyunsaturated margarine
(milk-free)*
⅔ cup honey
½ teaspoon vanilla essence
1¼ cups wholemeal self-raising flour
2 teaspoons baking powder
½ teaspoon cinnamon
1 teaspoon ground ginger
1¼ cups oat bran
½ cup soy drink
2 tablespoons finely chopped green ginger
1 egg white

METHOD

1. Preheat oven to 250°C (475°F).
2. Prepare a muffin tray by spraying with cooking spray.
3. Cream margarine, honey and vanilla.
4. Add remaining ingredients except egg white and mix well.
5. In a separate, clean, dry bowl, beat egg white until stiff and lightly fold into mixture.
6. Place tablespoons of mixture into prepared muffin tray.
7. Bake for approx. 12 minutes or until golden brown and cooked when tested.
8. When cooked, remove from oven and leave in tray for 5 minutes before placing onto a fine wire rack to cool.

Makes approx. 12 muffins.

MISCELLANY

	MILK-FREE	WHEAT-FREE	EGG-FREE	LOW-FAT	LOW-SUGAR	CONVECTION	MICROWAVE	FREEZER
Apricot Spread	•	•	•	•				•
Banana Smoothie	•	•	•	•				•
Chilli Sauce	•	•	•	•	•	•	•	•
Corn Relish	•	•	•	•	•	•	•	
Maria's Marvellous Taco Sauce	•	•	•	•	•	•		•
Muesli	•	•	•	•				•
Sweet and Sour Sauce	•	•	•	•		•		•
Tofu-Banana Cream	•	•	•					
Tofu Mayonnaise	•	•	•		•			
Tomato Gravy	•	•	•	•	•	•	•	•
Worcestershire Sauce	•	•	•	•	•	•		

APRICOT SPREAD

This is an alternative spread for bread. One tablespoon of the spread can also be used as a substitute for an egg yolk in a cake recipe. Fruit spreads are so named when they have no added sugar or artificial sweeteners.

INGREDIENTS
1 kg (2 lb) dried apricots
1 cup water
1 tablespoon concentrated apple juice
(no added sugar)

METHOD
1. Place apricots into a large bowl with a lid.
2. Pour in water and apple juice.
3. Seal and set aside for 24 hours.
4. Next day blend apricots and liquid in the bowl of an electric food processor or blender or rub through a sieve or Mouli.
5. Bottle in clean jars and seal. Store in the refrigerator until required.

Makes 3 x 375 g (12 oz) jars.

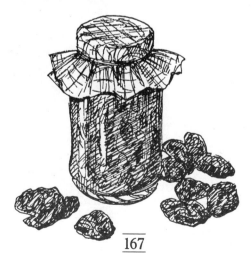

BANANA SMOOTHIE

This smoothie is a delicious, nutritious drink. It is made milk-free to suit a dairy-free diet. Best results will be obtained if the bananas are peeled and cut into small pieces and frozen overnight. The frozen pieces of banana are then used to make the smoothie. This smoothie can only be made by using an electric drink mixer of some type.

INGREDIENTS
2 ripe bananas, peeled and cut into small pieces
2 tablespoons soy drink powder
2 tablespoons ice-cream (see recipe page 130)
400 ml (13 ozs) iced water

METHOD
1. Place all the ingredients into an electric drink mixer and mix until very thick.

Makes 1 large serving.

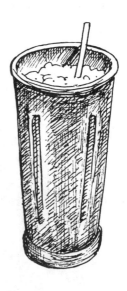

CHILLI SAUCE

This sauce can be served with lean meat of your choice or as an accompaniment to vegetable dishes. It has no added fat, sugar or salt.

INGREDIENTS
1 x 425 g can peeled tomatoes (no added salt)
2 tablespoons tomato paste (no added salt)
¼ cup white vinegar
2 tablespoons concentrated apple juice
   (no added sugar)
1 teaspoon dried oregano
½ teaspoon dried cumin
¼ teaspoon hot chilli powder (as desired)
½ cup chopped red pepper
1 small onion, peeled and chopped
1 clove garlic, peeled and crushed
1 x 425 g can baked beans (no added salt)

METHOD
1. Place all the ingredients into a medium sized bowl and stir well.
2. *Convection Cookery.* Place into a saucepan and simmer with the lid on for approx. 10 minutes, stirring occasionally.
or
   Microwave Cookery. Place into a microwave-safe bowl and microwave on high for approx. 5 minutes stirring occasionally.
3. Blend in an electric food processor or blender or rub through a sieve or Mouli.
4. Reheat and serve as desired.

CORN RELISH

This is a spread that can be used for sandwiches or added as flavour in dishes of your choice. It is a healthy recipe with no added sugar. It will keep in a sealed container in the refrigerator for 1 week.

INGREDIENTS
1 x 440 g can corn kernels (no added salt)
½ cup finely sliced celery
½ cup finely diced red capsicum
1 medium sized onion, peeled and cut
  into small dice
1 cup vegetable stock
2 tablespoons white vinegar
2 tablespoons maize cornflour
2 tablespoons concentrated apple juice
  (no added sugar)

METHOD
1. Place corn, celery, capsicum, onion, stock and vinegar into a medium sized saucepan or medium sized microwave-safe bowl and mix well.
2. Place cornflour into a small bowl. Blend with apple juice. Stir into ingredients in saucepan or microwave-safe bowl.
3. *Convection Cookery.* Stir over a gentle heat until mixture boils and thickens.
                    or
    Microwave Cookery. Microwave on high for 2 minutes and stir. Continue to microwave on high, stirring at 1 minute intervals until mixture boils and thickens.
4. Bottle into clean, warm jars and seal. Allow to cool and store in the refrigerator until required.

Makes approx. 500 g (1 lb).

MARIA'S MARVELLOUS TACO SAUCE

This is a very tasty sauce that can be stored in the refrigerator where it will keep for 1 week. It can be used for tacos and pizzas, for flavouring casseroles, or it can be served as an accompaniment with meals.

INGREDIENTS
2 tomatoes
1 clove garlic, peeled and crushed
1 small onion, peeled and cut into small dice
½ teaspoon hot paprika
2 tablespoons tomato paste (no added salt)
3 tablespoons concentrated apple juice
*   (no added sugar)*
3 tablespoons herb or white vinegar
½ teaspoon tabasco sauce
1 tablespoon maize cornflour

METHOD
1. Place tomatoes into boiling water and leave for 1 minute. Remove skins.
2. Blend all the ingredients in the bowl of an electric food processor or blender.
3. *Convection Cookery.* Place all the ingredients into a small saucepan. Stir over a gentle heat until mixture boils and thickens.

   or

   Microwave Cookery. Place all the ingredients into a small microwave-safe bowl. Microwave on high for 2 minutes and stir. Continue to microwave on high, stirring at 2 minute intervals, until sauce boils and thickens.
4. Bottle, seal and refrigerate until required.

Makes approx. 500 ml (1 pt).

MUESLI

Home-made muesli is not difficult or time consuming to make and is well worth the effort. If desired, muesli can be toasted on a flat tray under the griller. Care is necessary when toasting as some cereal ingredients can ignite easily. Allow to cool before storing in an airtight container until it is required for use. Larger quantities can be stored in the refrigerator or freezer for use at a later date.

INGREDIENTS
500 g (1 lb) rolled oats
¼ cup sesame seeds
250 g (8 ozs) rye or barley flakes
1 cup Sunfarm rice bran
2 cups natural dried fruit of your choice,
    e.g. sultanas or raisins
1 cup sunflower seed kernels
½ cup pepitas
½ cup chopped buckwheat kernels

METHOD
1. Mix ingredients together.
2. Store in an airtight container until required.

SWEET AND SOUR SAUCE

This sauce is easy to prepare and is suitable to serve with many foods, such as fish or veal, or it can be mixed into dishes for added flavour.

INGREDIENTS
1 teaspoon olive oil
½ red capsicum, seeded and cut into thin strips
1 carrot, peeled and cut into thin strips
1 small zucchini, cut into thin strips
1 onion, peeled and cut into thin rings
1 clove garlic, peeled and crushed
1 x 440 g can pineapple pieces (in natural juice)
1 tablespoon chopped green ginger
3 tablespoons concentrated apple juice
   (no added sugar)
1 tablespoon herb or white vinegar
3 tablespoons sweet white wine
1 tablespoon maize cornflour

METHOD
1. Heat oil in a non-stick frying pan.
2. Add capsicum, carrot, zucchini, onion and garlic and stir over a gentle heat for 3 minutes.
3. Drain pineapple and reserve juice.
4. Stir in pineapple pieces and ginger.
5. Mix together pineapple juice, apple juice, vinegar and white wine.
6. Place cornflour into a small bowl. Add a little liquid and blend well. Gradually stir in remaining liquid. Stir into vegetables and fruit in pan.
7. Stir until sauce boils and thickens.
8. Serve over selected food, or store in the refrigerator until required.

Makes approx. 3 cups sauce.

TOFU-BANANA CREAM

This cream is delicious to serve as a low-fat accompaniment to a dessert. The banana adds fibre and flavour to the recipe. The cream can be served as desired with any of your favourite hot or cold desserts.

INGREDIENTS
1 banana
200 g (6½ ozs) tofu
2 tablespoons orange juice
1 teaspoon finely grated orange rind

METHOD
1. Blend ingredients in the bowl of an electric food processor or blender, or rub through a sieve or Mouli.
2. Place into a small serving dish. Cover and refrigerate until required.

Serves 6.

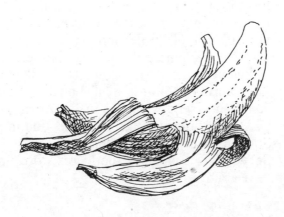

TOFU MAYONNAISE

This is an alternative mayonnaise for those who wish to follow a milk-free diet. Serve with salad or fish, or as desired.

INGREDIENTS

1 x 297 g packet soft tofu
1 small onion, peeled and chopped
1 tablespoon honey
½ teaspoon freshly crushed garlic
½ teaspoon cracked black peppercorns
1 teaspoon mustard
¼ teaspoon curry powder
juice of 1 lemon
1 tablespoon peanut oil

METHOD

1. Blend all the ingredients in the bowl of an electric food processor or blender until smooth (or mix together by hand).
2. Store in a sealed container and refrigerate until required.

TOMATO GRAVY

This tomato gravy can be used as a substitute for traditional gravy on lean meat, or it can be used as a sauce for spaghetti or other pasta. It is also suitable to use with fish.

INGREDIENTS
1 x 425 g can peeled tomatoes (no added salt)
1 small carrot, peeled and cut into small dice
1 tablespoon finely chopped fresh parsley
1 teaspoon dried mixed herbs (Italian variety)
1 teaspoon concentrated vegetable stock
2 tablespoons tomato paste (no added salt)

METHOD
1. Blend all the ingredients in the bowl of an electric food processor or blender.
2. *Convection Cookery.* Place into a small saucepan and cook over a low heat for approx. 5 minutes, stirring occasionally until gravy is slightly thickened.

   or

   Microwave Cookery. Place into a medium sized microwave-safe bowl. Microwave on high for 1 minute and stir. Continue to microwave on high, stirring at 1 minute intervals until gravy boils and thickens.
3. Serve in a gravy boat.

Serves 6-8.

WORCESTERSHIRE SAUCE

This is an easy recipe to make. You can store the sauce in a screw-top bottle for several weeks.

INGREDIENTS
500 ml (16 ozs) brown vinegar
1 small green cooking apple, peeled,
   cored and cut into small dice
1 teaspoon cayenne pepper
¼ teaspoon ground cloves
¼ teaspoon ground allspice
½ teaspoon ground ginger
1 clove garlic, peeled and crushed
1 tablespoon honey
1 tablespoon treacle

METHOD
1.   Place all the ingredients into a large saucepan.
2.   Stir over a low heat until ingredients are mixed.
3.   Simmer with lid on for approx. 1 hour.
4.   Rub through a strainer. Some of the sediment needs to come through the strainer as Worcestershire Sauce characteristically has some of the sediment in the bottom of the bottle.

Makes approx. 500 ml (16 ozs).

INDEX

179

Quiche
Carrot Quiche 92

Relish
Corn Relish 170
Rice
Brown Rice Salad 111
Butternut Rice 90
Fish and Spinach Rice 64

Salad
Brown Rice Salad 111
Cauliflower Salad 112
Cucumber Rings 34
Hot Bean Salad 113
Hot Potato Salad 114
Waldorf-Chicken Salad 115
Zucchini Salad 116
Salmon
Salmon Mould 70
Smoked Salmon Dip 37
Satay
Chicken Satay 54
Sauce
Chilli Sauce 169
Maria's Marvellous Taco Sauce 171
Sweet and Sour Sauce 173
Worcestershire Sauce 177
Slices
Marmalade Bars 149
Orange Slice 150
Sorbet
Apple Sorbet 126
Grape Sorbet 127
Lemon Sorbet 126
Orange Sorbet 124
Strawberry Sorbet 125
Soup
Cauliflower Soup 41
Pumpkin Vichyssoise 42
Tomato Soup 43
Tuna Soup 44
Zucchini Gazpacho 45
Soya Beans
Soya Bean Pizza 98
Soya Patties 100
Spaghetti
Spaghetti Bolognese 72

Spinach
Fish and Spinach Rice 64
Spinach Pâté 38
Strawberry
Strawberry Sorbet 125
Sweet and Sour Sauce 173
Sultana
Sultana-Grape Loaf 160

Taco Sauce
Maria's Marvellous Taco Sauce 171
Tofu
Tofu-Banana Cream 174
Tofu Ice-cream 130
Tofu Mayonnaise 175
Tofu Potatoes 110
Tomato
Tomato Gravy 176
Tomato Soup 43
Trout
Trout with Almonds 66
Tuna
Tuna Loaf 68
Tuna Soup 44

Veal
Osso Bucco 82
Veal and Vegetable Loaf 85
Veal in Red Wine 84
Vegetables (see also individual vegetables)
Beans Borlotti 86
Bean Casserole 88
Butternut Rice 90
Carrot Quiche 92
Carrot-Pineapple Cake 148
Cauliflower Salad 112
Cauliflower Soup 41
Chicken with Broccoli 50
Corn Bread 140
Corn Relish 170
Cucumber Rings 34
Fish and Spinach Rice 64
Garlic Zucchini 104
Ginger-Marmalade Potatoes 105
Honey-Ginger Carrots 106
Hot Bean Salad 113
Hot Potato Salad 114
Lamb and Vegetable Pie 78

Other Books published by the Author

Other Books in the Milner Healthy Living Series